# SAMURAI HEALER

## The Documented Story of How Cancer was Cured

By Adele Poenisch LLC

Edited by Patricia Givlin Dubrall
Endnote Research Assistance by
Amanda Remington

This book is published by ALIN Foundation Press LLC,
2705 Webster Street, #5885, Berkeley, CA (USA) 94705.
Orders may be placed at
www.alinfoundation.com

Printed in the United States of America

Library of Congress Control Number: 2025937426

Book design by Adele Poenisch LLC


ISBN: 979-8-21867195-2

# Dedication

To my parents Dorothy and Arthur Poenisch.
Thank you for your examples of honesty and courage.

To all the cancer therapy victims of the past three decades.

*Samurai History began in 1192*
*Samurai were Dedicated to Serve*
*and be Loyal to their Oath.*
*They Stressed Skill, Bravery, and a Moral Code,*
*To use Power with Discretion,*
*To be Honest in Word and Deed,*
*To Make Difficult Decisions based on their*
*Courage of Conviction,*
*To Act Correctly in Day-to-Day Interactions, and*
*To have Respect for others regardless of their*
*Status or Situation.*

# Table of Contents

# Author's Comments

*Samurai Healer* is both a reference library, and the story of a family and their love.

The endnotes superscript numbers point to information on the website www.Samurai-Healer.com. They document statements made in the book. As this book goes to press many endnotes, not critical to SEF™ claims, are still being documented. The website will always be a work in progress, and future editions of *Samurai Healer* will include new endnotes and point to their respective information. You can look at the research as you read, or you can read the book in its entirety and look at the research later.

Side Effect-Free Immuno-Chemotherapy™ cumulative result documentation is in the chapter titled **92% Long Term Remission of Terminal Cancers.** They can also be found in the peer review online periodical JMBio.org.

I greatly appreciate and want to thank Amanda Remington for her timely and thorough research that substantiated my many comments in this book. I also used endnotes compiled from ALIN Foundation research library, referenced valuable information from *The New England Journal of Medicine, Lancet,* and other reputable sources. Special thanks and great respect to Booking Institute and Health Harvard Education whose articles were invaluable in explaining the insurance and drug labyrinth.

Contact info@samurai-healer.com with comments or questions regarding this book.

If you need to inquire about Side Effect Free Immuno-Chemotherapy™ treatment go to www.Berkeley-Institute.com and submit an inquiry. You should receive a reply within 48 hours.

I have changed most names for privacy concerns and I've removed business names. I have tried to avoid HIPPA problems both in this book and in the endnotes at Samurai-Healer.com. A few real names were used in order to give people credit for their contribution.

I encourage you to do your own evaluations before engaging with any business or doctor.

I hope you enjoy and/or find the book interesting.

Adele Poenisch LLC

# Why You Need to Read this Book

The National Institute of Medicine reports "The lag between the discovery of more effective forms of treatment and their incorporation into routine patient care averages 17 years."

In response to this unacceptable lag, California passed Assembly Bill 592; an act to amend Section 2234.1 of their Business and Profession Code to say, "It is [therefore] prudent to give attention to new developments not only in general medical care but in the actual treatment of specific diseases...[1]"

Ya, ya, so it says...

The Google ad reads, "Don't give up hope until you've talked to us."[2]  So cancer victims apply, once conventional chemotherapy options have been exhausted, and they're only offered trials with a 50/50 chance of getting the placebo.  They apply, once the side effects from conventional chemo treatment make life not worth living.  They apply, when actuarial tables advise against payment.  And, they apply, because the shock of a terminal prognosis doesn't stop a person from wanting to live or from worrying about their family who must carry on alone.  Cancer can happen at any age to anyone.

Side Effect-Free [SEF, pronounced Safe] Immuno-Chemotherapy™ isn't a "sham" as the California Medical Board wants you to think when they revoked SEF Chemo™ developer Dr. Kenneth Matsumura's license December 8th, 2023.[3]  Greg W. Chambers, Supervising Deputy Attorney General, representing the complainants described Dr. Matsumura, whose 54 year medical record was unblemished until this case and who has 38 patents from his 63 years of medical research,  as "...cruel," that he "...was a liar," that he "...preyed upon...," and that his claims "...were delusional..."  These accusations were much more horrific than those made by the complainants.  But the December 1, 2023 San Francisco Chronicle carried Mr. Chamber's words to the public with the headline, "Despicable..."[4]

What did this "despicable" person do to bring down the wrath of the California Medical Board and Office of California's Attorney General?

<u>He invented a cure for cancer.</u>

Side Effect-Free Immuno-Chemotherapy™ eliminates the side effects of conventional chemotherapy. Those side effects are often worse than the disease. Many patients opt to die rather than continue conventional chemotherapy. But, without side effects, cancer victims can continue therapy until their cancer is gone.[5]

This makes SEF Immuno-Chemo™ an in-your-face direct competitor with conventional cancer therapy, and threatens the profits of hospitals and oncologists who treat patients and pharmaceutical companies who supply the medicines for cancer. A software programmer and early patient of Ken's interviewed for a job at a prestigious Bay Area university cancer center after SEF™ succeeded in putting his terminal bladder cancer into remission. The interviewer told him they make ALL their money from cancer treatments. Yeah, they don't make enough money from obscure maladies or treatable complaints. A hospital center does well to focus on cancer, the number two killer in the US.[6] Insurance willingly pays and passes on the cost for cancer therapies to all their policy holders. In 2023 alone cancer therapy generated 223 billion dollars of revenue for the health care industry. So the longer the therapy, and the longer someone can endure the therapy, the more insurance pays. Cancer is their bread and butter.[7]

There are many ways to die from cancer. Cancer is only one of them.

Shortly before the Medical Board revoked his license, Dr. Matsumura was treating among others, people who failed at Sloan Kettering Memorial, Stanford, Kaiser, and UCSF. He wasn't stealing patients. They found him and came when it became obvious their first choice, the popular choice, had nothing more to offer. He

2

was becoming known. He wasn't flying far under his competitions' radar anymore.

I am Dr. Matsumura's significant other. For the past 15 years, I've been amazed by a man whose singular focus has been on solving a problem for the benefit of mankind. It's past time to tell his story.

SEF Immuno-Chemo™ allows people to reach remission who are not just in stage 1 or 2 where growth has not spread beyond the originating organ, but in stage 3, when it has metastasized to a lymph node or in the case of lung cancer the other lung. It can even save those in stage 4 where cancer is all over the body, including the key organs, if those organs, liver, brain, kidney, and lungs, have not been compromised beyond their ability to rejuvenate.

When I talk to people about SEF Immuno-Chemo,™ when I explain its history of sending people with multiple types of cancer into long term remissions, when I tell them it is not uncomfortable because side effects from the chemo agent are minimal to none, they often exclaim in concerned surprise that they've never heard of it. If they've already gone through chemotherapy, they're especially dismayed.

SEF Immuno-Chemo™ was a promising therapy 31 years ago. In the 1993 FDA sponsored clinical trial at a major university medical center, pathology reports clearly indicated cancer cells were drastically reduced after one SEF™ treatment. Then in 2002 radiologists confirmed x-ray images showed SEF Immuno-Chemo™ had completely liquefied all the liver metastasis of one of Ken's significant relatives. In 2007 Ken achieved remission for four out of four terminally-ill clinical trial patients who had stage four breast cancer, terminal leukemia, and stage three B lung cancer.

Had his results been received with joy and excitement rather than contempt and jealousy, had team effort coalesced to speed SEF™ development rather than ignore his research and obstruct his progress, had SEF Immuno-Chemo™ been available to the public decades ago, one might wonder how many cancer victims would still be alive today?

# 2

For Ken his lonely journey to a cancer cure started decades before he lost his license and a lifetime before we remet. The journey traversed many paths, required numerous inspirations, and forced Ken to survive multiple financial and emotional hardships. Nothing curtailed his enthusiasm. Ken was focused on curing cancer. He decided this in high school.

He opened his medical research company, Immunity Research Laboratory, in 1961, when he was 15. As one of the top three students in Melvin Cavanaugh's Berkeley High science class, he was allowed to use Mr. Cavanaugh's back prep area for a lab. The science department head, Robert Rice, along with Mr. Cavanaugh both saw Ken's promise and arranged for him to do a fellowship in the Cancer Research Genetics Lab on the Berkeley Campus. There he met and worked under a renown cancer researcher, Kenneth de Ome.[8]  Mr. Rice also secured a grant for Ken making him the youngest grant recipient of the American Lung Association, formerly the Tuberculosis & Health Association and sender of Christmas Seals. To document his studies Ken wrote and self-published his first paper, "A Rapid Skingrafting Technique."[9]

Even with these demanding opportunities high school was easy. But grammar and middle school were challenging to a protected child new to America.

I think Ken's determination, his independent thinking, and his generosity come from his mother. Born in 1912 Vera was the second child of a Japanese family who were lured to the opportunities they heard about in California. In 1905 they settled in the large Japanese community in Alameda. Everyone attended the same Christian Methodist Buena Vista Church. At home her family maintained the traditional Japanese hierarchy relegating girls to secondary importance behind their brothers. Opportunities were not meant for everyone. But Vera couldn't be constrained by tradition. Her love of music drove her to practice piano on an imaginary keyboard under her bed covers. She was finally given a real piano when she was five and her destiny to become a concert pianist in Japan began.

She left California shortly before Pearl Harbor and the Japanese encampment and lived in Japan with extended family, until she met and married Ken's father. Shortly after the war the couple moved to Bangkok, Thailand where Ken was born in 1945. There, his mother gave piano concerts and his father worked for a shipping company.

Eventually, the family moved from Thailand back to Japan where Vera's popularity soared and Ken's father started making lots of money as the owner and designer of Homat Pre-fabricated Homes. The homes were designed to appeal to American GIs living in Japan. The Matsumuras lived in Takarazuka, Japan, in a very large Westernized home. But, unlike Western homes it had several maids and a chauffeur to take care of all the family's needs. Ken was pampered and spoiled. He was five when a wise "auntie" intervened to insist that he learn to wipe his own bottom. (An accomplishment he proudly told me about early on in our relationship.) Vera's life was socially and emotionally full.

It was 1955, in order to obey an over-zealous McCarthy Era citizenship requirement, Ken's mother, Vera, was forced to return to California from Japan to maintain her natural-born U.S. citizenship. Only Ken accompanied her. Once there she remained so Ken could get the American education both she and his father wanted for him. So Vera gave up the career she loved, her fame, her husband and, since yen couldn't be taken out of Japan, her wealth, in order to stay in America and raise Ken. Now piano students were her only means of support, and she taught out of their little studio apartment on Sacramento Street. But her ancestry included a samurai, of whom she was unduly proud, so defeat was not possible. For Ken the move was all those things, plus he had a new type of school and another language to learn. Good that he was *samurai* too.[10]

When Ken started grade school here at age 10, he weighed 58 pounds, so his classmates didn't worry about making fun of the little boy who tucked his shirt into his underpants. His 5th grade teacher, Mr. Albert Wells, stopped them with a warning to beware that this boy would someday do something great. Ken desired his teacher's confidence and readily participated during science class. When Mr. Wells made the statement, "Mammals don't lay eggs." Ken waved his hand enthusiastically. Fortunately, the veil of childhood parted just in time, and he was able to retract his hand, saving himself from a cringe-worthy flame-out when he realized the Easter Bunny is probably not scientific proof to the contrary.

Mostly though, the West Berkeley neighborhood his mother purposely chose for its multi-racial mix was accepting of all newcomers. Within three years their finances improved and they moved to a two bedroom house on Channing Way. While his mother gave her piano lessons, Ken, who is still bookish and quiet, liked to sit on the front lawn and gently pick up the honey bees that came by the thousands to collect pollen from the clover. He picked up hundreds of them, examining their little bodies, their cargo, and watching them socialize. One day a passerby asked Ken if he was afraid they might sting him. Ken had not known they could sting, and the next one he picked up did just that. It was a thought-provoking lesson. Do we really have enemies? Or does our fear make enemies? In facing the challenges in his life I've seen Ken choose multiple times, not to be afraid of danger. He is not naive. He carefully plans ways to avoid and minimize danger. But it comes because he's also not afraid to challenge the status quo.

The Channing house had one other great asset. My Grandmother lived next door. I met Ken when I was 9 and he was 12. My Grandmother Turner and his mother became best friends. His mother was 12 years younger than my Grandmother, which made her just a little older than a daughter my Grandmother had lost when she was just 19. Ken's mother used to ask my Grandmother for advice all the time and would often tell Ken that they should ask Mrs. Turner before they make a decision on something. My Grandmother loved Ken and always told us how smart he was. I can vaguely remember Ken inviting me to come over to his house to see the mice he was raising. I also remember wondering afterwards why he never asked me to come over again. He told me years later he used to watch me go up the stairs at my Grandmother's house, but was too shy to ask me to do anything with him because his mother

6

had told him what a special girl I was. That I was sweet and kind. He didn't think he was good enough.

We think they may have tried to "make a match-up" when I was 24 and he was 27. A very short meeting was arranged, and I always kid Ken that had he not just honked when he came to pick up his mother at my Grandmother's apartment things might have been different. Instead we just saw each other at the curb and said an awkward hello. I thought he was strikingly handsome, not the boy I remembered. Unbeknownst to his mother, he had already met and fallen in love with Molleen.

Years later, after my Grandmother died, I used to drive to Berkeley to visit with his mother. I was single, and realized the importance of friends. Vera's marriage had not weathered her separation from Ken's father. While they never divorced she was basically single most of her life. I'm sure she always missed my Grandmother. She used to give me delicate little Japanese gifts. One was an exquisite Japanese porcelain vase with two cranes on it. I later learned cranes mate for life and pairs are often depicted on marriage tapestries and dishes. Ken said he had wondered what happened to that vase because it was a treasured family heirloom. Well, now he has it back.

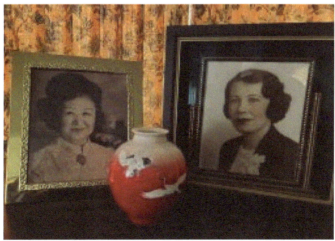

*Ken's mom, vase, Grandma Turner*

7

While Ken was still a teenager, he and his little company, Immunity Research Laboratory, were already engaged on the front lines of many medical battles. Cancer research was only one of them. He imagined and modeled himself to be like his idol, Thomas Edison, but for medicine rather than electricity. Inventing has always been Ken's greatest love. But his generosity and love of humanity has been what motivates him to invent. He wanted to solve humanity's problems.

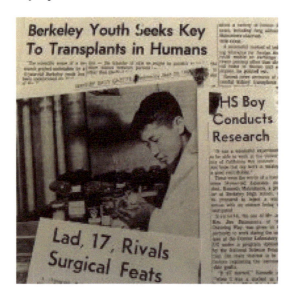

In high school Ken developed a methodology for making animal organs and tissues lose their transplant specificity so they can be transplanted from animal to animal or even animals to humans. He began to develop a method of growing kidneys, livers, and hearts in small table-top factories he called orplants, and registered Orplant American,[11] a business to sell organs for transplantation. He developed methods for blocking immunologic rejection of transplanted organs by causing what he called "immune paralysis." This technique overwhelms the ability of an animal's immune system to reject foreign grafts of organs.

Dr. Lola Kelly of Donner Laboratory in Berkeley became intrigued with his ideas on immune paralysis when they conversed during dinners at her father, Alexander Raab's, home. Mr. Raab was a well known pianist and friend of Rachmaninoff. He often hosted the local community of Berkeley musicians. Ken is a musician like his mother. Although, faced with his screaming objection in Ken's early years, she must have prevailed when insisting he practice piano at least two hours each day. By college, his piano coach, Peter Jarrett, tried to convince her Ken should be a concert pianist. But she was also practical and decided there was no economic future in concertizing. Although he no longer performs professionally, Ken still entertains himself and his family with beautifully expressive pieces by Rachmaninoff, Chopin, and his own compositions. The musician dinners did afford him another opportunity though. Dr. Kelly invited him to work in her laboratory under a second fellowship.

At the time of his transition from high school to UC Berkeley he thought both rejuvenation and a cure for cancer were pipe dreams. But he never abandoned hope they could become a reality in his lifetime. Today, with data from patient lab reports and testimonials from patients with terminal cancers to prove SEF Chemo's™ efficacy, he plans to turn his attention to our rejuvenation, more commonly called the Fountain of Youth. He is current on the work done by others, and has reasoned, but not yet contributed, possible solutions to the problems they are dealing with.

As a CAL Berkeley undergrad Ken continued his research fellowship on the immune system and skingrafting between 1963 and 1966. Dr. de Ome encouraged Ken to get a Ph.D, but Ken wanted to work with human patients directly, so passed on that suggestion to focus on medical school to get his M.D.

Near the end of Ken's third year at Berkeley, New York Life Insurance gave him a full scholarship to UCSF Medical School. The awarding representative later told Ken, she had never encountered anyone so unemotional when told they had just received a scholarship that would pay all medical school expenses, including room and board. He just said, "Thank you," and got off the phone.

Ken is calm.  He compromises and adjusts when the issue is not important.  He is immovably stubborn when he has reasoned why something should be his way.  His delivery and demeanor do not fluctuate much between elation and misery.  I envy his ability to always get that perfect night's sleep.

# 4

Side Effect-Free Chemotherapy™ was not imagined until 1984 well after Ken had graduated from UCSF and completed his residency at Kaiser.  He was attending a lecture for "Continuing Medical Education" credits, when his mind wandered, and he mused about how fairy tales usually involve a hero and a poisoned princess. The hero would come and save the princess by giving her the poison's antidote.  With that thought, his mind tripped from daydreaming into the realm of inspiration...if he preferentially delivered the poisonous chemo agent's antidote to normal dividing cells before administering the chemo agent itself, normal dividing cells would be protected, but dividing cancer cells would not.  He realized this was the answer to curing cancer.

"Chemo drugs" are chemicals that kill multiplying cells that are dividing anywhere in the body.[12]  If you take these drugs; you kill cancer cells.  But you also kill normal dividing cells, and, therein, lies the problem of conventional chemotherapy.

When chemo drugs kill stomach lining cells, patients develop nausea and vomiting. When they kill intestinal lining cells, patients develop diarrhea.  When they kill cells in the bone marrow, which makes red blood cells, patients become anemic and weak. When chemo agents kill the immune system cells, called white blood cells or neutrophils, patients aren't protected from infectious bacteria and can succumb to infections like pneumonia and meningitis.

To make matters worse, normal cells often divide more frequently than cancer cells, subjecting normal cells to greater lethal effects from chemo during the 48 hours after a chemo treatment remains in a patient's body.  For example, intestinal lining cells can divide every 24 hours, while lung cancer cells may divide only once in 72 hours. So one treatment with a chemo agent can kill two or three normal cells before one cancer cell is killed.

Ken felt chemo agents did effectively kill cancer cells, but patients could not stand the side effects. So they would often voluntarily chose to stop a chemotherapy that might have been curative, and explain their decision to their doctor with, "No more, please...this isn't life." Ken reasoned that if normal cell destruction could be substantially eliminated, more patients would opt to continue chemotherapy, and more would have a better chance of being cured. Chemo agents for most cancers lacked complete efficacy, and many patients would still die, especially, if their cancer had spread too far. But lessening side effects would enable patients to continue chemotherapy longer. So eliminating side effects would still save or lengthen many lives, without making the patients miserable in the process.

One of the hurdles to ordinary chemotherapy's effectiveness is side effects so severe that doctors can only administer their therapy every three weeks. To enable treatment every week or every two weeks doctors have to reduce the chemo dose, but that limits efficacy too, and the patient gets the same sad result. Normal cells don't over populate, plus many are lost just performing their daily duties. Cancer has no size restrictions or daily duties to curtail its growth. The three week delay between treatments gives cancer a great recovery advantage. Ken's approach of protecting normal dividing cells with an antidote changes the schedule to the patient's advantage, and when desirable, Ken can administer full dose SEF Chemo™ weekly.

There are medicines that can lessen the symptoms of the nausea and fatigue conventional chemotherapy chemo agents cause.[13] But true health will always depend on having a sufficient supply of normal cells to perform bodily functions.

Where cells are in their division process determines how susceptible they are to being maimed or killed by a chemo agent. During many phases of division the chemo agent's impact may only make a cancer cell sick. The cancer cells that survive the initial chemo treatment figure out or "learn" ways to protect themselves

11

from that agent the next time. Subsequently, their offspring, created through cell division, are also resistant to the same agent. To remedy this doctors move onto other, often more toxic, chemo agents.

If conventional chemotherapy patients persevere through the treatment, their original cancer, a ball of abnormal body cells that divide and multiply without control, morphs into a ball of body cells that divide and multiply without control, AND is resistant to every chemo agent available. Then your oncologist will tell you they have no more drugs, and offer you hospice care until your body fills with these abnormal cells, and you die.

Up until this new approach of using an antidote dawned on Ken his research laboratory at One ALIN Plaza in Berkeley had spent hundreds of thousands of dollars over 15 years following the theory that the best way to get rid of cancer is by identifying some unique chemical or marker on the surface of the cancer cell not found on normal cells.[14] But by the early 1980s he began to doubt this would ever produce a cure. There are different variations of cancer cells in every tumor. Out of a thousand cancer cells 990 may have the identified unique marker, but 10 may not.[15] While it might be possible to devise a way to kill the 990, those elusive 10 would remain alive. They would multiply, and their new generations would end up killing the patient. Ken was the only medical researcher willing to cast aside the time and money he had already invested and admit the theory of targeting cancer cells, the primary theory directing cancer research today will never work. Conventional chemotherapy's "Emperor has no clothes."

# 5

When Ken began to test out his new approach in the laboratory using an antidote during chemotherapy, he was puzzled to observe that his approach not only reduced side effects of chemotherapy, but made the chemotherapy more powerful and efficacious. Like a good scientist, he didn't believe the initial results. But when animals and, especially, in 2006 when his four phase II clinical trial patients, who all tested as having hopeless cancer, got well, Ken began to look for an explanation.

It was nearly a decade before he realized his addition of an antidote made his therapy also immune therapeutic, not just chemically therapeutic. By using an antidote he observed the body's immune white blood cells or neutrophils, cells typically decimated in ordinary chemotherapy, were, somehow, preserved. These neutrophils were enabling the killing of more cancer cells. It wasn't necessary to increase the chemo agent. Neutrophils appeared to be augmenting chemo's power, making it like chemo on crack cocaine.

Neutrophils divide rapidly. They protect us from harmful bacteria that cause infectious diseases like pneumonia and meningitis. Like the honey bees Ken gently examined as a boy, neutrophils give their all to do the job of killing invasive germs and getting rid of old, dead and injured body cells. They must be constantly replenished by the bone marrow. If neutrophils are destroyed by a medication, such as chemo, the bone marrow which produces them cannot replace them fast enough to clean up the mess. Besides being prone to infection, the patient is left with a feeling of fatigue due to the overload of dead and dying normal and cancer cells cluttering their body. Unfortunately, in conventional chemotherapy neutrophils are killed along with everything else dividing.

SEF Immuno-Chemo™ protects neutrophil cells so they don't get sick or killed. They remain healthy and available to do the jobs they were designed to do. Three types of neutrophils cells work as a team to do a job called the Neutrophil Cascade. The first type travels around to find the aged, sick or injured cells — cells just like the cancer cells that get bombarded with the chemo agent. It marks them. The second pummels these marked cells until they are thoroughly tattered and torn up. Then the third dissolves [phagocytize] the beat up cells so they can be carried away by the blood for disposal through bodily processes.[16] After a SEF Immuno-Chemo™ treatment neutrophils are still there to immediately go to work.

This second wave of killing was a complete surprise to Ken who was only aiming to control side effects of chemo. Bravo to our immune system. I have to estimate here as different cancers have different results. But also destroying the injured cancer cells probably doubles the number of cancer cells killed in one treatment.

Combining our unaltered immune system with SEF Chemotherapy™ created the only therapy in the world effective enough to eradicate cancer within a reasonable number of treatments. Because SEF Chemo™ is chemotherapy plus immune therapy.

# 6

Several years ago, I argued with Ken to change the name from SEF Chemo™ to SEF Immuno-Chemotherapy.™ Especially, since even google search engines recognized our website as the only "neutrophil potentiated" cancer therapy. But at the time he thought the 85% failure rate other scientists were experiencing with their version of immune therapy gave it too much bad press. Not only was immune therapy often not working, it sometimes left behind permanent horrific side effects.[17] One of Ken's patients, a 32 year old woman, came to Ken after a German immune therapy was unable to stop her breast cancer. She was responding well to SEF,™ but side effects from her previous immune treatment caused fluid to pool around what had been her healthy heart. She had to be admitted to the hospital during COVID because of these side effects, and overworked ICU staff allowed a hydrating tube to flood her lungs. She left behind a husband, a three year old daughter, and a mother who will never recover from losing her.

Currently, so-called "immune therapy" research focuses on a different immune cell, called white blood lymphocytes, not neutrophils. Scientists extract a patient's white blood lymphocytes and place them in a test tube. There, outside the patient's body, they try to teach the cells how to attack the patient's cancer. Sometimes this works, often it doesn't, more often than not there are serious side effects and sometimes cancer growth is even accelerated. Immune therapy, like conventional chemotherapy, tries to identify a cancer cell by a unique marker or protein on its surface. But each type of cancer has different markers, so immune therapy must be tailored to a particular cancer type.

However, a famous immune therapy success was former President Jimmy Carter, whose melanoma skin cancer, diagnosed in 2015, metastasized to his brain. After receiving immune therapy, he reached remission in 2016. But again, targeting cancer cells, as immune therapy does, does not eradicate cancer. At 98 in 2022, Carter came out of remission and opted to enter hospice care, rather than seek further treatment for his cancer. He died peacefully shortly after his 100th birthday in 2024.[18]

I understood and accepted Ken's reasoning, but I believe it was unfortunate that we did not change SEF Chemo's™ name. Had we done so, the Medical Board might have had to acknowledge that SEF Immuno-Chemotherapy™ is unique and truly an alternative medicine. Instead they ignored the California Business and Professional Code Section 2234.1 that says "A physician and surgeon shall not be subject to discipline pursuant to subdivision (b), (c), or (d) of Section 2234.1 solely on the basis that the treatment or advice he or she rendered to a patient is alternative or complementary medicine,..." Ken presented evidence of proper (b), (c), and (d) subdivisions. The code goes on to define "'alternative or complementary medicine' means those health care methods of diagnosis, treatment or healing that are not generally used but that provide a reasonable potential for therapeutic gain in a patient's medical condition, that is not outweighed by the risk of the health care method."[1] Since SEF Immuno-Chemo™ uses a completely different immune system blood cell, neutrophils, not lymphocytes, it is different from both ordinary chemo and the immune therapies others are developing. I believe the California Medical Board was in error to judge Ken's therapy as poorly executed ordinary chemotherapy.

Regarding other immune therapies currently underdevelopment, maybe it's audacious to attempt to change our immune system, and test this methodology on people when medical science does not yet understand nor has it yet been successful in treating autoimmune diseases. Thank goodness, 10-15% of those treated for cancer do benefit from their lymphocyte immune therapy. But is a 10-15% success rate really enough "...therapeutic gain..." to merit the FDA's approval and insurance coverage when side effects include death?

Ken's SEF Immuno-Chemo™ reaps the benefits of our immune system naturally. While he uses conventional chemotherapy chemicals for SEF Immuno-Chemo,™ he doesn't need to change our immune system nor use immune system altering drugs and chemicals. Because SEF Immuno-Chemo™ protects the immune system from the chemo agents, the neutrophils remain healthy and can attack and dissolve cancer cells injured in a chemotherapy treatment. Ken invented SEF Chemotherapy,™ an entirely new Side Effect-Free cancer therapy. But by using SEF Chemo™ he discovered SEF Immuno-Chemotherapy,™ an even more powerful Side Effect-Free cancer therapy.

The Medical Board refused to consider SEF Immuno-Chemo™ as an "alternative or complementary medicine." They compared it to only chemotherapy and brought in chemotherapy expert witnesses to examine the defense Ken presented. Of course their experts' experience did not prepare them to evaluate immuno-chemotherapy. The test results, test scheduling, treatment schedules, and protocols Ken presented he learned over the last 18 years as he treated or supervised treatment of patients in his four clinics. Ken's patients' needs and their test results were different and completely new to the chemo experts' training and to their thinking. Rather than admit that they did not have similar experience, they claimed he deviated from "standard of care" and misrepresented test results. No consideration was given to the testimonies from his cancer patients, who had been diagnosed as terminally ill by their oncologists, and have now returned to their normal routines while quite alive.

Below is an example of the extreme brevity Judge Juliet E. Cox took when writing the court order.

At the trial one terminal-cancer survivor treated with SEF Immuno-Chemo™ testified,

"...Taylor MD my Urologist Oncology Surgeon did another follow-up check and said that in his 30-year career he never saw anything like this and all the multiple tumors in the bladder were all gone. Matsumura MD... continued monitoring me along with Taylor MD for over 5 years without any cancer recurrence. Today, I am still in complete remission after over 7 years."[19]

In the order the judge summarized his entire statement as,

"He believes himself currently to be cancer-free."

Besides drastically reducing the number of cancer cells by killing the injured cells, SEF Immuno-Chemo™ prevents injured cells from recovering and making generations of cancer cells resistant to the chemo agent. Without this resistance, Ken's therapy is able to primarily use only one chemo agent, carboplatin. Ken chose carboplatin because it is one of the most effective and potent chemo agents available. Conventional chemotherapy typically uses carboplatin a lot in desperate situations because its side effects can be so severe. But with SEF Immuno-Chemo™ large carboplatin doses can be given without the patient suffering at all.

The side effect of hair loss is definitely a morale buster. Hair is expendable so follicles divide rapidly, and hair falls out constantly. Ken could not create a test for hair loss so he doesn't make claims. Carboplatin is one of the chemo agents that does not induce much hair loss, and his patients, even when Ken uses another of the several agents he's tested, have not reported loosing their hair. Some have claimed their hair became darker and thicker. I suspect we can all deal with that!

# 7

As Ken neared puberty, Vera asked a gentleman friend what she should do to raise her son to be a man. He said, "Make him do everything." From 12 years of age on, she gave Ken all the responsibility needed to run their little household. She herself was a savvy investor and once enthusiastically told me, "I love the stock market. I love it when I win. I love it when I lose. I love it." And rightfully so, as she studied it and did well. Had I taken a few of her suggestions, I would be richer today.

From age 12 on Ken made their financial decisions, including buying a house and car. Today Ken does his personal and company taxes without advisors or software. After a nine month IRS audit he owed nothing. The agent concluded the audit by asking him how his artificial pancreas work was going. His investments and what he made as a doctor financed his research. He's never received money from government programs nor has he become indebted to venture capitalists. It was natural for him to open one business and register another while still in high school and finish UCSF medical school and his residency at Kaiser by age 26.

Having grown up wealthy he was conservative, and considered himself aligned with Republicans. With a Japanese-American mother, Japanese father and Thai birth, three governments could have drafted him. Fortunately, he had renounced his Japanese and Thai citizenship and done well in school. He started CAL Berkeley in the fall of 1963, the year before the Free Speech Movement started.[20]

Originally, the movement centered around a topic Ken had frequently discussed with his friends. The disparity between rich and poor. William Knowland, publisher of the Oakland Tribune complained to his friend, CAL Chancellor Ed Strong, about CAL students protesting his paper's employment policies outside his newspaper and on the CAL campus. However, those policies took advantage of many of the paper's employees who were also CAL students. To placate his friend, Strong wrote a new campus policy saying students were no longer allowed to distribute political fliers. They were here to get an education. His edict changed the movement's intent. Student leaders objected, saying this policy denied them their right of free speech. Ken could see they were not making bizarre demands.

800 students were arrested, including leaders Ken thought were quite reasonable. Berkeley was all over the news. My grandmother

from Iowa called my Mom to ask if my sister, a freshman chemistry major at Berkeley, was OK. When asked, Donna complained that police helicopters had disrupted her final. So much for that education Strong purported to serve.

By now, Ken was participating in about every demonstration, but kept a low profile. He was heading to medical school with hopes of becoming a doctor and didn't want any publicity that might be negatively construed.

Ken saw that the press slanted the issues towards Knowland and Strong's viewpoint,[21]and made the protesters and their issues appear extreme and irrational. Through editorials and by omitting facts the press framed the cacophony a communist movement.

Knowland and Strong also used their money to influence decision makers in the California State legislature who then supported their actions. Ken now saw how news content and policy were beholding to contributions. Until he experienced this blatant bias, he believed working hard with good intentions would eventually solve world equity problems. The poor would get their due. But it was clear that without money the poor would never have justice. No one would hear their side, and their lives would not improve. Demanding the right to speak freely is important because unseemly messy protests are the only way the injustices of the poor will ever be heard.

Ken does not begrudge the rich their wealth, but believes they should recognize it as the result of the efforts of many, not just theirs. Their wealth was earned through contributions made by people they knew, by people they never knew, and by people long dead. In humble acknowledgment of these contributions the rich need to use their money to make the world better for everyone. In Ken's enormous capacity to empathize, he felt the suffering of the poor as his personal responsibility to solve. He designed his life's plan to create a better world. Not only would his inventions improve humanity's health, but the money those inventions generated would be his tool to improve society.

# 8

During his formative undergraduate years, Ken came up with the idea of creating a foundation-corporation. Not a non-profit, but a for-profit company focused on public service. He felt any industry like transportation, medicine, energy, utilities or production of food that affects the welfare of humans should not be purely for-profit. In addition he wanted his company's profit to be "value-added profit." That is profit produced from his and others' creative endeavors...not "exploitative profit" made from the depletion of resources or people or a people. In 1971, he renamed his Immunity Research Laboratory ALIN Corporation-Foundation International.[22] The acronym ALIN originated from the words artificial liver. He would go on later to create ALIN Foundation Institute,[23] a 501(c)3 public benefit entity that can be found at ALINfoundation.com. The tax status was an after thought and only used once.

Initially, the focus of his public benefit entity was education. He created a small publication called, "*BASE – A Journal of Science & Technology,*"[24] where high school students and college undergrads could publish articles explaining their discoveries and ideas. Normally peer reviewed journals demand people have an academic position at a university. Without such a position the important discoveries of students either remained unknown or had to be credited to their academic advisors, who were able to publish. Ken solicited professors at universities to "peer review" the articles he received. These professors advised Ken whether the articles were worthy of publication, and Ken published the best. Together Ken and his old teacher Robert Rice created a science board that included such illustrious notable as Carl Sagan, Nobelists Glenn T. Seaborg, and David S. Saxon, MIT Chairman. Around year 1999, *BASE* was renamed *Science21Magazine.* The hard copy publication was discontinued and replaced by www.science21magazine.org. The new name included the number 21, which referred to the century just ahead. It was meant to invite the reader to take a peek at the inventions of the future, and meet the young new minds who would shape it.

Around 2016 Ken created another scientific periodical. The *Journal of Medicine and Biology* can be found at JMBio.org where qualified scientists can instantly publish.[55] JMBio's innovative design allows literally thousands of peer scientists to review and criticize submissions. This approach is considerably superior to how other journals operate. Submissions to other journals are reviewed by only a handful of scientists and their comments do not accompany the article they reviewed. This limited reviewing still takes between 6 and 15 months, delays publication until it's complete, and results in bias. Today, when open discussion is demanded and rapid results expected, a delayed publication method that harbors closed opinions is archaic. JMBio's publication process, called Metprex,™ (Met means change, and prex means publish) opens up peer reviewing to thousands of scientists, with differing ideas, not necessarily the "standard" ones.

JMBio is an open forum, but with qualifications to publish or review. A scientist must have published at least 3 articles in another periodical or can be sponsored by a qualified scientist. Its key innovation is "post-publication peer-review." Once accepted, authors and reviewers can upload their articles or reviews for immediate publication. Degree initials are not to be included in a submission for publication. This practice hearkens back to the days when reviewers did not depend on the letters behind names to judge an idea. Conflicts of interest must be revealed. Public peer review can be embarrassing so submitters tend to be extra careful in what they write. More criteria and instructions can be found at JMBio.org.

Like economics and politics, even experts have a variety of opinions. Medical journal editors decide which articles are published and which are not. Therefore, articles about cancer and its treatment can be limited to what supports the editors' preference to one belief or methodology.

I have gone into detail regarding "peer review" journals because it seems they have become "influencers" wielding authority beyond the likely merits of the few people who decide what scientific innovations the world will hear about. At Ken's 2018 press conference,[25] due to this "peer review" mystique the nightly news

21

reporter inadvertently slanted her viewers acceptance of SEF Immuno-Chemo.™ At the end of her announcement she said, "he has self-published." She didn't even include the JMBio website, so people could read it for themselves. Nor did she say that his article was peer reviewed.

Ken still enjoys sharing his excitement for science with young people. In the Fall of 2023 he ran a two day lab experiment with the three sons of one of his patients. Since Sandy was a patient during COVID Ken made numerous trips to her home in Turlock, California. He became very close with her entire family, and trained her 15 year old son, Jason, to administer several therapies to correct her potassium level and help her platelet count problem. He trained her mother to perform the basic duties of a nurse, including tracking and dispensing the necessary prescribed medications. While Sandy responded well to SEF Immuno-Chemo,™ it became clear she had a undiagnosed competing malady, immunopathic thrombocytopenia.[26] Sandy's mother remembered her daughter as having been prone to frequent and prolonged bruising throughout her childhood, but never dreamed it was a life threatening disease. Thrombocytopenia is a rare autoimmune disease that causes low platelet levels, and platelets are needed for blood clotting. Even though she had had two pregnancies (one single and a pair of twins) her condition was evidently not apparent to her obstetrician. As an internal medicine doctor, Ken identified it immediately. It was obvious from the sustained bruising where tumors had died that her platelet level was not sufficient to clot her blood. What would have been a successful cancer outcome was thwarted by an incurable disease. While in the ICU to remedy her low platelet count, the nurses were too busy during COVID to turn her. When she returned home her back was covered in bed sores that refused to heal. The family and Ken decided not to readmit her. Sadly, the boys lost their mother to breast cancer coupled with an autoimmune system disease and inadvertently to COVID in 2021.

The two day teaching lab Ken conducted with the boys was to test the potency of chemo agents Ken doesn't use but may use in the future. The Medical Board had accused Ken of padding his bills by adding an unnecessary charge for chemo agent potency testing. But Ken thought it was necessary. Years before he discovered the carboplatin, produced by several reputable pharmaceutical companies, had lost some or all of its ability to kill cancer before its expiration date. This meant that conventional chemotherapy patients' cancer advanced while they still suffered the side effects of the weak chemo agent. In 2007 Ken reported his findings to the FDA, but never heard back. Ken's teaching lab has not yet reached a conclusion. Regardless, Ken tests all the medicine he uses for its potency before giving it to his patients. Ken believes the FDA is diligent ensuring only fully potent drug leave the factory, but they don't have policy on how drugs are transported and stored. Some drugs could get stuck on a hot Texas tarmac inside a plane waiting to take off. Ken's advised me never to sign up to have my prescriptions delivered, but to pick them up at a pharmacy.

I suspect his most ardent sharing was with his daughter, Marjorie. In 1986 when Marjorie was eight, Ken wanted to pique her interest in the sciences. They worked together on an experiment using mice to prove the validity of the basic concept for Side Effect-free Chemo.™ They were simply making sure there were no side effects from chemo when good cells are protected with an antidote. Nine times out of ten experiments reliably fail. But to his amazement, and I'm sure, Marjorie's innocent expectation, the experiment was a complete success. It was even more impressive than expected. This was long before he had used SEF™ on a human patient, and he recognized the phenomenal breakthrough would be indicative of future successes. Their experiment was not meant to to encourage his daughter to become a doctor. He just wanted her to respect and trust the scientific process. It was already obvious to him the medical world was changing. Insurance and government payers were dictating how patients should be treated. Financial considerations took precedence over his preferred "Dr. Marcus Welby" style of care. Marjorie, happy to work with her sweet Daddy and duly impressed, did follow in his footsteps but towards his social justice goals. She is currently a California director of a non-profit 501(c)3 organization that weaves strategic alliances

23

between labor, neighborhoods, housing, and other organizations to build people power.

## 9

When we re-met in 2010 Ken told me of his dream to enrich the poor. He explained how SEF Immuno-Chemo™ worked and showed me his treatment results. I was truly puzzled. Like most people, I couldn't understand why the medical world hadn't already embraced it. Why was the world still suffering from this horrible disease? Why were people still enduring the side effects of chemotherapy, when SEF Immuno-Chemo™ protected their good cells so there wouldn't be side effects? When I was out for walks or we were driving I would think, "I'm so lucky to know cancer is cured. I'm not like people I see walking around me or driving in other cars. They still worry whenever they have a routine doctor appointment that something horrid might be discovered. They believed the specter of cancer was still a threat." I was sad they weren't relieved of this worry. If only, they too knew. It took me awhile to see and understand how the hurdles of market competition fortified with hostile blacklisting, false reviews, and online hacking had stifling Ken's enrollment and his dreams for an equal society. Only patients already skeptical of conventional chemotherapy and looking for alternative solutions inquired. Fewer took the leap of faith and enrolled in a therapy "outside the box."

I'm susceptible to marketing ploys and advertising as much as anyone else. Even though like many Americans I've read *Hidden Persuaders*, I can succumb too easily to consensual thinking, trends and behaviors. I used to feel most comfortable going with what has been "tested" by popular demand. But I learned the hard way that group thinking can lead to big mistakes, not just in purchases, but in life's major decisions. Breaking from the norm is hard. Both mine and Ken's best friends opted to get conventional chemotherapy when they were diagnosed with cancer. Fortunately, neither were very sick. We're happy they did what they felt most comfortable doing.

My friend is still alive, but Ken's friend's cancer is progressively getting worse.

We tried to connect with various people who were famous enough that news covered their cancer diagnosis. We sent FedEx letters to Joe and Jill Biden when their son Beau had brain cancer, to President Hugo Chavez of Venezuela when he had some sort of abdominal cancer, and to Shannon Doherty before she died of breast cancer. We never heard back from any of them. Once he was no longer in politics, I successfully connected through Facebook messaging with Harry Reid, former Senate Majority Leader. I explained SEF Immuno-Chemo™ to him. He seemed interested and asked if I was a doctor. I said, "No, though I know a lot about this therapy." I also warned him we were badly hacked. For several days we continued our conversation. Then one morning his entire Facebook page was deleted and all entries he had made to my Facebook account were erased. Sadly, he never contacted us, and later died from pancreatic cancer. I'm sure he continued to go to the "best" doctors. But no other doctor, except Ken, using SEF Immuno-Chemo,™ has a history of putting pancreatic cancer like Reed's into long term remission. Following the norm should not be seen as a decision. At best, it's someone else's judgment, and their decision. As popular as it might seem, it may not fit you at all. Using your own best judgment, and questioning our current medical protocols is not only prudent, it may be lifesaving.

## 10

Even though Ken remains without huge sums of money, it is his nature to intervene and help individuals when he can. I've watched him actively solve immediate issues for many. But I believe, his greatest gift was showing them he acknowledged their self-worth. It is also how I fell in love with the sweetest person I ever met. I consider myself brave and I believe I persevere, but his bravery and continuous generosity is astounding. Two of the next three accounts are my own. The first Ken told me.

A homeless man settled into the alley adjacent to the front door of Ken's Dwight Way office building. Things became a mess, and Ken's employees and renters complained. Ken approached the man and simply asked if there was someone he could call for him. Immediately the man rattled off a phone number. When Ken called, the woman who answered screamed. She yelled to her husband, "My God, they found John!" After getting the pertinent information she said crying, "We're leaving immediately. It will probably take us three days." They would drive continuously from Kentucky. John was her husband's brother and father to their nephew, who, out of necessity, was living with them. John had been a successful tree surgeon in Kentucky. But after a bad fall he was crippled and unable to work. His life spiraled down and he was too disoriented to remedy his situation. He drove to Carmel, California and then to Berkeley, where rents were not affordable. So he started living in his Mercedes, until it was confiscated by the Berkeley police. Living in a car is against the law, while living on the street then was not.[27] Ken called an ambulance and told John to tell the hospital he couldn't walk so they would admit him. At the hospital, to avoid shocking his family, they cleaned him up. Three days later all were happily united. For the next 15 years while John remained alive, Ken received Christmas cards from the family updating him on John's renewed life.[28]

John's story may just seem lucky, since it resolved quickly, but the majority of Ken's caring involves years of unfailing conviction that the person was capable and deserved a better future.

Sara, our beloved family member, is called "Auntie" by Marjorie's children and "daughter" by Ken. Sara came as a refugee from the Balkan Peninsula at age 12 to live with a wealthy family in the Highlands neighborhood of Berkeley. She and Marjorie became close friends at Masterson-Bates High School, and soon Marjorie was inviting her home on a regular basis. In casual conversation Ken and Molleen came to understand Sara was not having a social life. As they had always wanted a large family, it was natural for them to emotionally adopt her. Happily, they included her on vacations, excursions, dinners out, and her achievements were recognized and celebrated. Though her parents are still alive Sara calls Ken Pa, and referred to Molleen as Ma. Ken meets with her parents whenever they are in the Bay Area. A surrogate sister to Marjorie and consummate aunt to Marjorie's two children, Sara never misses a family birthday or celebration. Fortunately, she has settled close by with her husband. We love them both.

West Oakland Health Center gives medical help to the poorest. When Ken started there in 1971 he didn't expect to stay 45 years. But he did. One of his patients, a young business executive, was looking forward to celebrating her first year of sobriety, and trying to get back on her feet. But she was unemployed, homeless, emotionally agitated, and unfamiliar with being poor. Her $400 shoes did not wear well on the sidewalks. Her embarrassed Tiburon parents had abandoned her. One of Ken's investment properties was vacant so he housed her there...for 5 years. When she emptied her storage unit during move-in she was too distressed to function and couldn't hang up the tangled ton of expensive clothes. I helped her. Once settled in she began to stabilize. Ken employed her as best he could to fit his business needs. Two years later she met her future husband at an AA meeting. He moved in, and soon after got a job. Near the end of the five years they married, and before their first child was born, moved near her sister in Seattle. Having gained back her confidence and finding happiness, she was offered an executive job out of state. From there she has continued to excel in her field. She still sends us family videos of their children, and we watch her life continue to unfold.

So the poor need money. But they also need acknowledgment to gain self-respect and confidence to seek out and accept opportunities. They need a safe space, and they need time to recover. Poverty can happen to anyone because anyone can have an accident, emotionally break from pressure that leads to self-medication and addiction, or live where there is political upheaval. It is often not an individual's problem or failure. It's just life. While many would like to frame poor people as ne'er-do-wells or worse as criminals, they're humans, deserving of respect and consideration first and accusations only if truly culpable.

Ken likes money. He believes money is needed for a modicum of personal comfort. Today, due to centuries of disparity, he believes money's main purpose needs to be to re-balance our society. Those who want to be listed by Forbes Magazine may end up the richest people in the world, but money is a low bar when it comes to what you could aspire to do to make your life valuable. Ken sees money not as the goal, but as a means to do good because he thinks it can be the most powerful tool to help people be their best selves.

The Free Speech Movement in 1964 influenced Ken's plans for his life. He knew he was given talents and he wanted to use them to make the world better for everyone. He hoped to create opportunities, so all people could realize their life's meaning and feel happiness. In the fifteen years we've been together he hasn't had money. But that hasn't stopped him from helping individuals. His frustration is that his dream has always been bigger than that.

## 11

Ken's Immunity Research Lab started in a high school back room, then moved with Ken to a CAL Berkeley cancer lab, but in 1967 when he started medical school at UCSF he relocated his company to his mom's house in Berkeley. Even though his scholarship paid his room and board at UCSF he returned home each night to tend his experiments and to walk, Alex, their dog. At UCSF he continued testing and perfecting his methodology using skingrafts to prevent transplant rejection. He became very proficient and was able to do a dozen skin transplants in a minute. But Ken's interest was also piqued by the work of other scientists who were busy experimenting with a new idea of placing skin tissue inside a small semipermeable container. They kept the tissue alive with the nutrients and oxygen carried by blood they passed across the container's surface.

His life was busy, but each day back in Berkeley he was able to relax. One warm evening, while walking Alex, the two of them were able to access a creative plane only dogs and their masters experience. Ken can still feel that moment on Magnolia Street, its houses, their porch lights. When he thought, if he could use some tissue other than skin, maybe kidney or liver cells from an animal organ inside the container, they would be protected by the container's semipermeable surface, and immunological lymphocytes would not be able to cross into the container and kill the cells. With that revelation, he knew he had invented a bio-artificial liver.

He hadn't been trying to invent an artificial liver. No one thought it could be done because the liver is so complex that all its functions remain unknown. It is known that the liver detoxifies poisons such as the ammonia our bodies make while metabolizing. Without the liver these poisons would render us comatose. The liver also makes and delivers to the bloodstream vital molecules that keep the mind sharp. Beyond that our liver remains a mystery.[29] So no one was trying, and certainly not student Ken, to invent an artificial liver. Even though it would only be a temporary fix for a person in liver failure, a bio-artificial liver would allow that person to live while their liver rejuvenated. Passing the blood from the person via an infusion tube across the semipermeable surface that encapsulated liver cells in a bio-artificial device would off-load liver duties, and neutralized the body's poisons, giving them the time their liver needed to heal.

Ken continued his unsupervised studies using artificial organs at the same time he was in medical school. By modifying the semipermeable material with one of a larger porosity, he found he could encapsulate pancreatic islet cells instead of liver cells. When blood with elevated levels of sugar indirectly contacted the pancreatic cells, insulin at the precise amount needed to lower sugar blood would be released by the pancreatic cells across the semipermeable material into the blood. Once normal blood sugar level was reached the adding of insulin to the blood would automatically stop. At the time the best attempts of other researchers only measured blood sugar levels with a device that would automatically add insulin from a reservoir into the bloodstream if sugar levels were high. But Ken recognized that such a cumbersome mechanical process was fraught with all kinds of dangers when used for such a precise and delicate function.

# Artificial Liver Invention Claimed Here

By AUGUST MAGGY
Gazette Staff Writer

A young Berkeley physician-scientist has developed what he says is the world's first artificial liver.

The announcement yesterday by Immunity Research Laboratory of Berkeley, a private research organization, is expected to startle the medical world.

The artificial liver called a hepatic support device has undergone successful laboratory tests and will be tested on human soon.

DR. K. N. MATSUMURA, 29, educated at the University of

...here and Berkeley High School, stressed that the device is still strictly experimental and hoped none of its development would not generate any "false hopes" among people suffering from liver ailments.

The young doctor, who has been associated with Immunity Research ever since the lab was established here more than six years ago, developed the artificial liver over a period of seven years research work in the field of organ transplantation.

He began his work at the assuming use of it.

He said the device, which duplicates almost all of the functions of the complex human liver, was developed with some "several pigs."

"CERTAIN ACCIDENTAL discoveries" led to the device's development, he explained.

The artificial liver is about the size of an average book and weighs two pounds.

The new device is designed to be used intermittently unlike the human body like the artificial kidney by passing diseased blood from the patient's limb through the device and returning treated blood to the patient.

The device is designed as an economically produced and disposable unit.

"THE DEVELOPMENT OF an artificial liver has always been believed to be virtually impossible because of the liver's

(Turn to Page 2, Col. 7)

## Berkeley Daily Gazette

For 92 Years the Home Newspaper of the Greater Berkeley Community

BERKELEY, CALIFORNIA, SATURDAY, JUNE 27, 1970    No. 155    10c Per Copy—$2.25 per Month

WEATHER
Fair Sunday. Low clouds along coast extending inland night and mornings. Low in the 50s, high near 80 along coast to 90s inland. Winds to 20 mph.

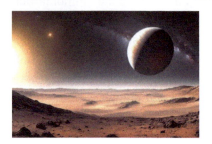

Matsumura bio-artificial pancreas manufactured in zero gravity of Outer Space

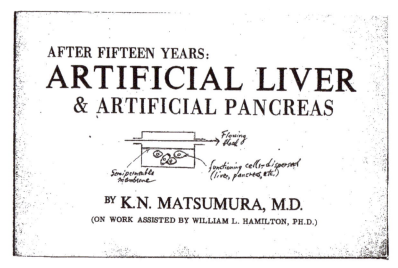

AFTER FIFTEEN YEARS:

# ARTIFICIAL LIVER
## & ARTIFICIAL PANCREAS

BY K.N. MATSUMURA, M.D.

(ON WORK ASSISTED BY WILLIAM L. HAMILTON, PH.D.)

*J&J and Ken worked together to use the Artificial Pancreas in zero gravity outer space.*

30

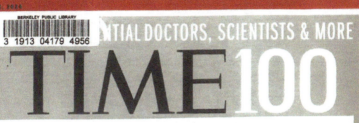

## ...NTIAL DOCTORS, SCIENTISTS & MORE

# TIME 100

## Artificial Liver - Best Inventions of 2001

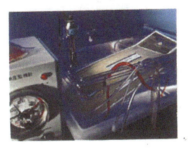

### Inventor: Dr.Kenneth Matsumura, Alin Foundation

The liver is one of the most complex organs in the body. It removes toxins from the blood and manufactures up to 1,000 proteins, metabolites and other vital substances. Now scientists trying to develop an artificial liver have found a way around these complexities: they let rabbit-liver cells do the work. The Bio-Artificial Liver developed by Dr. Kenneth Matsumura has a two-part chamber—patient's blood on one side, live rabbit cells suspended in a solution on the other—with a semipermeable membrane in between. As toxins from the blood pass through the membrane, the rabbit cells metabolize them and send the resulting proteins and other good things back to the other side. Because the rabbit cells never come into direct contact with human blood, the chances of infection or rejection are minimized. The device will support a human while diseased liver regenerates.

*TIME recognition of Artificial Liver.*

Ken filed for patents on both his bio-artifical liver and bio-artifical pancreas. According to his patent attorney, these were granted in record time of a few months.[30] The news spread on the second and third pages in newspapers worldwide. Of course, The Berkeley Gazette[31] put it on the front page. Ken got lots of letters from everywhere. Brown University announced it was creating a brand new laboratory dedicated to research using bio-artificial devices. Now bio-artificial devices are called hybrid organs, and progressive years of research have produced hybrid kidneys and even vaginas.[33]

In 1986 Johnson and Johnson, the largest healthcare company at the time, asked Ken to collaborate on a pencil-like device that would contain pancreatic islet beta cells surrounded by a tubular semi-permeable membrane. These would be slipped into the abdominal fat pads of diabetic children who were self-injecting insulin four times a day. He worked with Jack McConnell, Executive VP and second in command at J&J,[34] the two of them planned to manufacture the bio-pancreatic devices in anti-gravity inside the space shuttle. Although Ken was hesitant about shuttle technology, he appreciated the chance to save the lives of millions of children who without such a device would age fast and many die in their thirties. Unfortunately, the Space Shuttle disaster ended the project. Dr. McConnell was devastated as were all Americans, and the project was abandoned.

In 2001, thirty years later, the idea for the bio-artificial liver was recognized by Time Magazine as one of the inventions of the 2000 decade,[35] and Ken was given credit. By then it was being copied worldwide. Young people in liver coma from viral hepatitis were being saved. Iran published articles on their version. Except for the Time Magazine shout out, almost no one mentioned where they got the idea. Such is the fate of inventors and their patents. Unless, like the inventor of the intermittent speed windshield wiper you want to spend your life defending a patent, it's really the manufacturers and those who sell inventions that reap monetary benefits.

# 12

Ken has not gotten rich on his inventions, but lack of wealth didn't dissuade him from his goal of eliminating the disparity between rich and poor. Upon finishing his residency at Kaiser, and opening his private practice specializing in diabetes in Berkeley, he answered the call to serve in America's poorest ghetto, West Oakland. In 1969 President Johnson's National Health Service[36] started funding medical centers in each ghetto community across America. Until these centers opened, the poor had only county hospitals to go to. At 7 AM they would arrive at the hospital, get a number good only for that day then wait and wait. At 4 PM many had not been seen and were sent home. The determined repeated the process the next day hoping for better results, but most gave up and let their diabetes and hypertension get worse. Each ghetto received five million dollars from the National Health Service to create a health center. These centers then invited the community physicians to donate some of their time serving the local poor.[37] With doctors available it was hoped the clinics could schedule appointments and eliminate the insanity of pointless waiting. Ken was paid about one quarter what he made at his private practice, but he stayed because he saw that these people didn't come in unless they were really sick.

All but two clinics for the poor opened under Johnson's National Health Service plan exhausted their funding within a couple years. West Oakland Health Center (WOHC) was one of them. It remained solvent because of a black man named, Robert Ray Cooper. Dr. Cooper was born in Alexandria, Louisiana. His family moved to California in 1947 where he attended public schools in Alameda county. He graduated from CAL Berkeley in 1955 and received his M.D. from UCSF three years later. Two years after that he completed his internship and residency in pediatrics at the Alameda County Highlands Hospital. He remained at Highlands becoming their Deputy Director of all medical training programs, while also running his private pediatrics practice in Berkeley. About 1970 Dr. Cooper started at the West Oakland Health Center as Chief of Pediatrics under Section 330 of the United States Health

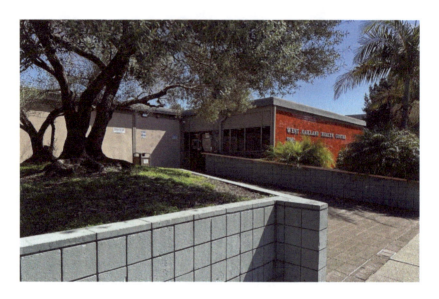

Resources and Services Administration (HRSA) grantee. This grant was funded to provide a broad range of health services to under served primarily indigent residents of West Oakland. Dr. Cooper was the best thing that ever happened to the West Oakland Health Center.

Ken started at West Oakland shortly after Dr. Cooper. By 1972 it was becoming obvious that ghetto centers were running through their funding. The five million which was suppose to last five years, had been given to and was managed by community ministers. Ministers are often not experts versed in the "bread" part of living. They had never seen so much money and hired every brother, sister, cousin, and auntie. Their workers lined the halls of all the beautiful new health centers, but without the proper skills they were unable to attract patients, or manage and replenish their coffers. In West Oakland the "volunteer" physicians asked the National Health Service to be allowed to run the health center, and in 1973 WOHC physicians appointed Dr. Cooper the Health Center's Executive Director. Shortly thereafter in response to their favored status, he completed his MPH in Health Planning and Administration from the School of Public Health at CAL Berkeley.

By federal law WOHC was required to provide services to its patients for a fee determined to be affordable according to their household income. Less than 10% of the patient population could be billed the full cost of service fees. Of those billed only 20% paid the fees. Regardless, with toughness and skill and deflecting all pressure, even death threats, Cooper balanced the books. No small part of that balance was due to the resilient WOHC physician-volunteers. As their Director of Urgent Care, Ken handled all after hours healthcare. The pay was so poor that Ken kept as an example two checks totaling $3.68. These he received as MediCal's adjusted payment in lieu of the $76.00 bill he sent them to cover a 4 hour 2 AM house call.

Unfortunately, Ken sought a reference letter from Dr. Cooper after the Medical Board hearing. Ken's attorney had not asked for references. His attorney felt that the Medical Board and State Deputy Attorney General Chambers had made so many errors in adjudicating Ken's procedures and SEF™ therapy that it would be an easy win. He said he had successfully won similar cases of Complaint Investigation by presenting them as alternative therapies, and cited CA bill 592. But the previous experience he had that warranted his $650 per hour charge, did not prepare him for the corporate-medical "machine" he was up against, and he lost the Medical Board hearing in August 2023. He asked to be excused from service and for Ken to pay what remained due of his fee. Ken filed his own appeals in 2024, but was defeated on technicalities. He is now in the process of taking his case to the U.S. Supreme Court where he will again represent himself.

I include quotes from Dr. Cooper's letter here. As Ken's superior, Dr. Cooper's letter represents authoritative knowledge of Ken's performance from 1971 to 2013 (42 years.) It holds precise testimony that can defend Ken against several of the prosecutor's incriminating accusations used by Judge Juliet E. Cox to support her verdict.

Dr. Cooper wrote,

"Dr. Matsumura records were periodically reviewed by internal staff and representatives from federal, state, and city and met the specific documentation standards designed to protect to the extent possible all entities from significant liability for malpractice incidents."

"I know Dr. Matsumura's records were never a cause of concern as regards standard compliance."

He continued,

"I know he [Ken] did not complain about the amount of the fees charged or the percent of the fees actually collected. I also know that his patients complained less about his services than they did about other providers and that he provided patient oriented and disease outcome directive, being very adamant and direct and refusing requests for narcotic pain relievers and [instead] promoting healthy diets. I know that a number of patients may have perceived his refusal to provide "strong pain medication" and his bluntness regarding the promotion of healthy diets as cruel."

Dr. Cooper closed by saying,

"I was pleased to have him as member of the WOHC staff and am willing to so testify under penalty of perjury if asked or required to do so."

Judge Cox wrote her order using only words from the prosecutor and complainants. She ignored the plethora of carefully written medical notes on patients, including Ken's notes saying a patient's tumor shrank and became barely palpable after SEF™ treatment. She ignored a statement by a patient under treatment who said she felt well enough to leave her SEF™ therapy. She believed instead, the Medical Board's comments that Ken had not presented anything about this patient's care. She discounted all correspondence that showed he carefully presented other alternative treatments, including expected outcome from SEF Immuno-

Chemo™ [3] as compared to the expected outcomes with conventional chemotherapies.™

Relying on fifteen hours of court time, she cast judgment on 63 years of a man's life when she wrote:

> "[Physician]... is exempt from discipline only if the physician surrendering this treatment [SEF Immuno-Chemo™] has secured the patient's consent to the treatment after giving the patient complete, accurate information both about conventional treatments for the patient's illness and about the potential risks or benefits of the "alternative or complimentary" treatment....respondent did no such thing. Rather, he gave his patients and their families wildly inaccurate information about the potential benefits and risks of the treatment he offered, about the benefits and risks of other available treatments, and about the patients' own conditions."

> "A physician's failure to maintain adequate and accurate patient care records is unprofessional conduct...with respect to patients 1,2, and 3...constitut[ing] cause to revoke respondent's [Ken] physician's and surgeon's certificate."

For those undergoing SEF Immuno-Chemo™ Ken finds extra strength acetaminophen [Tylenol] quite adequate to ease the pain of even his stage 4 cancer patients. Reading the transcript from the hearing and the experts frequent reference to "standard of care" I was reminded of a conversation I had with a woman who told me after her cataract surgery the hospital offered her fentanyl. When she hesitated and asked if another medication would also work, they said, "Yes. You could use Tylenol." In light of our current pain management aka opioid epidemic in the U.S., I have to wonder if not using narcotics was the underlying problem they were really alluding to when they said Ken was not performing "standard of care."

## 13

WOHC received most of its money from Medicare and MediCal, California's version of Medicaid. Both were created in 1965 under the Johnson administration. Medicare subsidizes health care payments for disabled and citizens over 65. MediCal subsidizes those payment for qualified poor. A few WOHC patients did have private insurance, but they were rare.

At WOHC Ken saw that Medicare's new payment systems were prone to abuse. His observation has proven true, and we are now all aware of how the flaws in Medicare and its influence on private insurances have festered. Soon after its start, hospitals and doctors recognized that as long as they uniformly increased their prices Medicare would pay because that increase could be passed on in the form of higher private insurance premiums and national debt. This caused our country's health care annual cost, plus the interest paid on the debt it created, to increase from 38 billion before 1965, when many patients paid out of pocket, to 4.5 trillion in 2023.[40]

There needs to be lots of discussion on how to solve our ginormous health care costs, but here are a few of the ideas Ken shared with me. Basically, he believes patients need to retain the right to scrutinize their health care. They should be able to contest their bill, like any person does when they hire a contractor or buy a product.

With patients scrutinizing their own bills, the costly billing monitors that Medicare and insurance companies have hired by the hundreds of thousands since 1965, at the cost of billions of dollars, would become obsolete. Hospitals and doctors would think twice before sending their patients a bill charging $20 for a disposable bedpan or $200 for a six minute office visit because they'd know they would lose that patient's business. Insurance companies and their billing clerks would no longer be the ones who decide yea or nay to allow or disallow a drug or medical procedure that may determine the quality of your life. You and your doctor would decide whether a procedure was worth the cost. Competition would drive down the prices, rather than working in partnership to raise them.

If you worry about unemployed billing monitors. Don't. Insurance companies hire the best and the brightest. Medicare billing monitors, who lose their jobs, are highly qualified and should be able to easily change to other, hopefully more useful occupations.

Ken believes hospitals and doctors need to attract patients in the good old fashion way with competitive pricing and good quality care. He still wants the government to continue subsidizing health care, but suggests allocating a certain amount of health credit annually to each citizen. Sort of a government funded Health Savings Plan. If the credit is not used, it would accumulate. It could also be shared or donated, and passed along in a will. Expensive or chronic medical problems would probably need special funding, and would have to rely on the general public or large groups of people. Possibly similar to what is offered to members of the Church of Latter-day Saints should one of them be injured while offering their services to the church.[42]

Competitive pricing would make patients conscious of budgeting, and hospitals and practitioners would have to give them an estimate of the costs prior to a treatment. Then patients could compare the estimate to what is considered "normal" for that treatment. Like price matching between Lowes and Home Depot, their favorite doctor might even be willing to lower his estimate. In fair turn-around, patients who constantly haggled and/or didn't pay would soon find no one wanting to treat them. Debit cards carried by each person would include immediate approval amounts for emergency services.

On the provider side, the billing monitors that remained would take on new tasks. Besides billing and giving estimates to patients they would identify marketing possibilities, cost inefficiencies, and relay situations or practices that create unhappy customers. Patient complaints would have consequences for the hospital or doctors because the free market would be grading them, like it does for elective care now, and used to do before 1965.

As people begin to again feel empowered and in control of their health care cost, I'm sure more adjustments would be forthcoming, similar to California's 2022 AB35 bill, which corrected the MICRA malpractice lawsuit cap enacted in 1975. AB35 changed the maximum malpractice reward from $250 thousand to $750 thousand, an amount to be phased in over a period of 10 years. Hopefully soon, a correction will also be made to the statue of limitations for malpractice. A year is not enough time for patients or family members traumatized by a flawed medical procedure to regain their composure and file for malpractice. Optimistically, we might hope, patient scrutiny would also result in fewer malpractice issues.

## 14

In addition to after hours care at WOHC, around 1980 Ken took over all In-Patient Services and began admitting all patients needing to go into hospitals. He felt he had more patients in the two Berkeley hospitals, Herrick and Alta Bates, than all the other internists combined. But around 1983, during Reagan's first term, the U.S. Congress amended the Social Security Act to include a national Diagnosis-Related Grouping System[41] for hospital payments. This meant patients could only stay in the hospital a certain number of days depending upon their diagnosis. So a diagnosis of pneumonia might be given 2.3 days of hospital care, regardless of whether the patient's age was 25 or 90. Initially Ken tried to avoid discharging his patients who were still too ill by hiding from the utilization nurse in stairwells and the bathroom, but he soon realized he needed to protest this draconian edict by denying hospitals of income and not admitting any patients. This also meant denying himself the income from hospital visits, an amount slightly more than he received for an office visit. He took voluntary admitting leave[43] and hoped other physicians would do the same. Nationwide they could stop the DRGS payment system. Forty years later, contrary to statements made during his hearing implying he is prohibited from admitting patients, Ken is still on voluntary leave. To date no other physician has joined him.

Ken's early political action that had the most impact towards balancing rich and poor was raising the minimum wage for Californians. In 2005 when California Governor Arnold Schwarzenegger twice vetoed a bill to raise the minimum wage from $6.75 to $7.25,[44] Ken was incensed. He was knocking himself out trying to keep the working poor he served in West Oakland healthy, but his patients often told him they had to cut their medications in half to make it last until their next payday. Taking half their needed amount made it impossible to control their hypertension and diabetes. Often they couldn't fill their prescriptions at all.

In the Fall of 2005 Ken started a recall Schwarzenegger movement and organized 10,000 volunteers to circulate and get signatures for a ballot initiative. Many were members of the Democratic Executive Committee of California. He created a website www.SaveCalNow.com where he posted daily reports of their progress and demands. On Sept 28 he held a press conference where he announced the recall campaign. Schwarzenegger's job rating was already down to 30%. Ken swears Marie Shriver Schwarzenegger was reading the website and relaying it to Arnold because in Arnold's consecutive speeches he kept modifying his views to match the movement's demands. In November 2005 Schwarzenegger hired a new Chief of Staff, Susan Kennedy, of no connection to the Kennedy family, a Democrat and important worker for climate and LGBTQ rights. But that did not satisfy Ken. He continued the pressure by publishing the Recall Campaign's Platform criticizing how Arnold ignored California's infrastructure, how he was messing up on water distribution between North and South, and how it was important to legislate cuts in carbon production. Ken's interviews on CBS and ABC radio aired statewide. Besides a minimum wage increase he was now campaigning on climate issues. Fighting fire with fire, Ken purposely chose and started talking with actor Warren Beatty and his spouse actress Annette Bening for the Recall Campaign's gubernatorial candidate to replace Schwarzenegger.

By January 2006 Schwarzenegger said in his State of the State of California address, "the one thing he wanted most was to raise California's minimum wage.[45] In June that year the emboldened legislature sent him a new minimum wage bill for $7.50."[47] In September he signed it into law to give California's poor the highest minimum wage in the nation. Before year's end he signed legislation to curb green house gases. Obama copied California's climate laws for the feds.[48] In December of 2005 Ken's "daily note" on his website had identified the recall's demands. Schwarzenegger's November 2006 re-election campaign platform was designed to address the entire list. Out of his fear of being recalled, Schwarzenegger had remade his policies and his image.

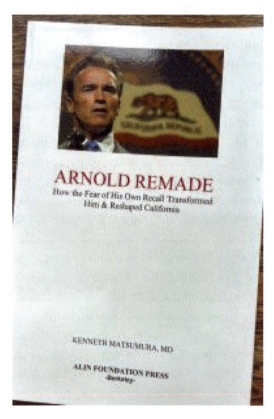

*Available at ALINfoundation.com*

Realizing he had achieved his goal, Ken wrote a grateful farewell book to his volunteers for their successful effort, *Arnold*

*Remade: How the Fear of His Own Recall Transformed Him and Reshaped California.*[46]  With Ken's perseverance and determination they had delivered $5 billion to the working poor and into California's circulating economy.  They had also initiated valuable climate solutions that continue to protect our nation today.  For Ken it was an experience that proved one person could make a big difference.

# 16

Berkeley's mild weather and proximity to research and manufacturing hubs of the greater San Francisco Bay Area meant consistently rising real estate values.  Ken loves Berkeley and we seldom venture far outside the surrounding area.  His roots here are as deep as the Redwoods are high.  The convenient great real estate was the perfect opportunity to fund his research.  Rather than go to venture capitalists or seek bank loans, he bought and developed property then leveraged it to access cash.

As a teenager Ken spent summers in Tokyo with his architect father where he learned real estate development and architecture. His father, Jiro Matsumura, along with Miss Keiko Showa, his father's business partner, provided luxury Western style homes to wealthy executive American and Europeans working in Japan. Between the time Ken separated from his father at age 10 and these summer visits, Homat Homes, his father's business, had become a million possibly billion dollar company.  Ken cherished these visits, and they became very close.  He loved his father dearly, but in 1970 when his father sought a divorce, Ken, an only child, felt obligated to side with his mother.  Vera was adamant.  She was still very connected to her relatives and friends in Japan.  She didn't want nor deserve the stigma a divorce would cast on a Japanese woman. Japan did not have "no fault" divorces.  After a heartbreaking fight it was Ken who provided the final proof that his father was the one who abandoned the family.  His father disowned him.  Even though, Ken had invented his Heart Attack-Alert Watchwrist™ his father did not have one when he died from a heart attack in 1988 and left everything to Miss Showa.

After we re-met, in an attempt to heal the past, Ken wrote to Miss Showa to say he now understood how loneliness and human need can drive people together. He told her how he now loved and was very compatible with someone new. Sadly, Miss Showa never replied. I believe the emotional wound Ken carries of his father's disappointment never healed, and he quietly remembers and pays tribute to him by using the skills his father taught him: developing, refurbishing, renting, buying and reselling in Berkeley.

Ken's largest and most successful investment property started when he sub-leased from Dwight Hardware their run down retail space a block away from downtown Berkeley. Dwight Hardware wanted to vacate before their low cost 20 year lease was up. As a sub-leaser Ken was able to sub-sub-lease the space at the higher rate being asked on the cross street, Shattuck. This enabled him to cover Dwight Hardware's obligation to the land owner plus clear $6,000 a month. He used the proceeds to improve the property and took profit.

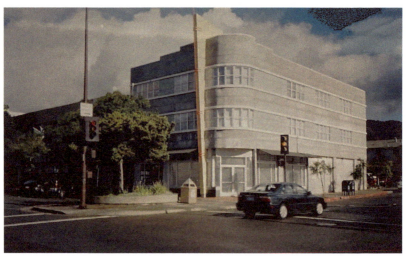

*One ALIN Plaza*

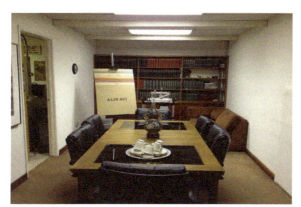

*ALIN Foundation Headquarters Conference*

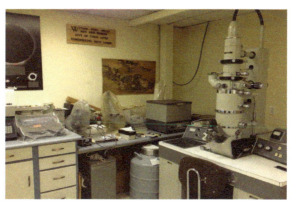

*ALIN Research Facility*

Then, estimating the land owner would soon be interested in selling, Ken bet 80 thousand dollars he had in savings to renovate a building he didn't own. His intuition was right. The owner died, and his family sold Ken the property for $399,360 a price appropriate for an old building with a low rental rate potential. Further financing was easy, because Ken had equity in the improved property. The sale included an adjoining undeveloped near acre parcel. Once he was owner he added a two story 2,000 square foot building on the North East side increasing his property value and his rental income. A few years later he borrowed against that investment, and built a 15,000 square foot three story building on the Southwest corner of Shattuck and Dwight Way. This addition created a Gateway to Berkeley's Downtown. He renamed this sprawling corner property One ALIN Plaza, and used 10,000 square feet on the second and third floors of the corner building to house his research laboratory and corporate office. In 2002 the 2107 Dwight Way property value was estimated at 7.2 million.

## 17

At home, once Elly wasn't a baby anymore, Molleen became politically active and focused on protecting the teaching of evolution in schools. As a Secular Humanists Society co-leader with Paul Kurtz, she was head of the Evolution Studies at the National Center for Science education. In 1999 she successfully stopped a Kansas law that would transition teaching evolution to the teaching of Biblical creationism in the public schools. Her success had repercussions on similar efforts in Oklahoma and Texas. More information about her writings can be found in *Marquis' Who's Who in America,* and in *Pregnancy with Disabilities* a book she ghost wrote and published. Then online work was cumbersome and slow, but she

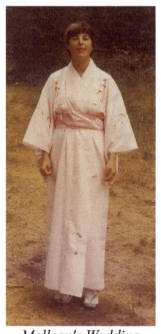

*Molleen's Wedding Day*

was productive. Her enthusiasm led Ken to start exploring online forums too.

They both found they preferred Prodigy to America Online or General Electric's Genie because the leaders or "hosts" for each topic or "forum" seemed more congenial. Other networks allowed

46

people to name-call and be highly critical of differing points of view. This circular finger-pointing never produced meaningful discussions or novel results. It usually ended up with discouraged people just dropping out of the group. Prodigy hosts encouraged people to compliment each other. Being in a Prodigy forum was ego healthy and usually thought provoking. Prodigy soon became the most popular early online network.

Ken started his own somewhat political forum titled, "Words Together." He coached his attendees to be respectful, to start counter comments with phrases like "I never thought of it that way" or "Well, you raise some interesting points, but have you thought instead…" His group congealed into many long distance friendships between disparate personalities. A young woman named Andy wrote a lengthy opinion of how poor people are discriminated upon. She said as an adult she still found it difficult to sever the monetary and emotional effects of her impoverished childhood. She pointed out it takes practice to grab opportunities, and poor people have few. She also reminded other forum members that potential can't be reached when basic needs aren't even met. Don, a wealthy, retired, mid-level executive from IBM, joined her discussion to argue his conservative view. Keeping within the forum rules their heated view points started with admiration and respect. So the sharp jabs stemming from prior pain and conviction dissolved in non-threatening discourse, and allowed the foundation for collaborative thinking to form. They were able to find common understanding, and both won: Admissions from Don, such as, "Andy, I never thought of it that way. Thank you for opening my eyes," and Andy's comment, "I thought rich people were just mean people, but I can see why they think in certain ways. I am learning." After a year of combative banter, Ken was amazed when Andy told Don, "You are the grandfather I never had." He loved it, and everyone on the forum started referring to him as "Grandpa Don." Today our social media revels in cruelty, and no one tempers it. But it wasn't always, and doesn't have to be run like the island kingdom of *Lord of the Flies*. "Words Together" demonstrated that admiration and camaraderie is more powerful than disdain and aversion.

Internet and cellular connections were still sci-fi. Anything online was through a modem using a telephone line. Prodigy announced they were losing tons of money because so many people were tying up their phone lines for hours while they wrote. This forced them to buy more and more lines so other customers could connect. They proposed charging an hourly fee. Ken admitted he was on between 4-5 hours, and Molleen, 6-7 hours a day. They'd easily have a monthly bill exceeding $200. A huge number of people were elderly shut-ins who couldn't make friends in any other way. Many were on fixed incomes, and a new discretionary expense was out of the question. Everyone started writing sad notes lamenting that they would be alone again. By that time, Ken was the impromptu "rep" for his Prodigy Users Group. PUGs championed complaints from Prodigy users who thought it important to keep the Prodigy platform user-friendly. Ken was pretty successful at getting their problems solved, and around two months before charging was to begin, his Words Together forum asked him to create a different Prodigy that wouldn't have to charge. He tried to laugh it off by saying Sears and IBM spent $100 million to create Prodigy. I don't have a fraction of that! And you want me to make something they couldn't. But then an idea occurred to him. Keep the people off-line while they wrote and have them just connect when they were ready to send. He would only need a few 800 numbers because people could just call, send what they wrote, download new messages, and hang up. Once off-line they could answer new messages on their personal computers. It seemed doable. But before hiring two programmers and spending his own money he asked his users to show their interest by sending him $39.90 for first and last month service. This minimum charge would pay for the 800 numbers they would eventually use. He doesn't remember exactly how many responded, but enough to convince him to go ahead. Within two months they had more than a forum. They had a new network, the "People Together Network," PTN.com. Then came an "ah ha" moment, 800 numbers allowed PTN to send and receive emails anywhere in the world, including for the first time supplying email service to rural America. America Online, Sears Prodigy, and GEnie couldn't, but PTN could!

Within a few years the popularity of the online forums diminished as the internet added more services. In addition, the Y2K date change was a hurdle too high for Prodigy, and it shutdown in late 1999. The new Internet could deliver news, and its embedded algorithms captured people's attention by verifying their opinions rather than encouraging discourse.

# 18

As consumers were becoming accustomed to using computers, Ken turned his attention to projects that measured bodily functions. One invention kept track of internal temperature and alerted the wearer when ovulation happened. Another gave an alert of a pending heart attack.

The Ovumeter pin-pointed ovulation allowing a woman to either get pregnant or avoid pregnancy. Tucked within a pessary, which was then placed inside the vagina, it accurately records temperature fluctuation throughout a woman's monthly menstrual cycle. The comfortable and discrete pessary could be worn for a year. It required little attention. To plan a family the wearer just had to watch the LEDS colors on a separate handheld display, red for no baby, green for baby, and yellow for maybe baby.

I laughed when Ken told me about the Ovumeter and thought the name much too scientific to entice a woman to use it. As a 12 year old, I can remember staring blanking at a sectional line drawing of half a woman on the Tampax instructions.[49] It was a sectional side view showing: one leg, vagina canal, uterus, and torso from stomach down. I had to wonder, "Where IS that on me?" So I was relieved when Ken readily accepted my suggestion to tone down the scientific rhetoric and rename it Egg-Timer.™ In June 2022 when the Supreme Court struck down Roe vs. Wade,[50] Ken and I briefly revisited the Egg-Timer™ trying to push it into production. But as legal issues with the State of California Medical Board heated up we had to abandon the effort.

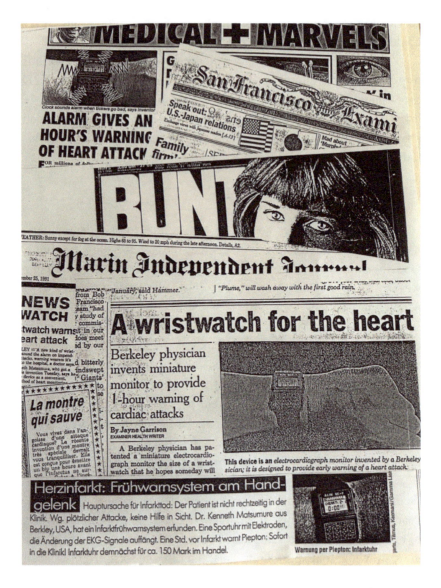

**MEDICAL + MARVELS**

*San Francisco Examiner*

Clock sounds alarm when ticker go bad, says inventor

**ALARM GIVES AN HOUR'S WARNING OF HEART ATTACK**

FOR millions of fol...

**BUN**

WEATHER: Sunny except for fog at the ocean. Highs 65 to 95. Wind to 20 mph during the late afternoon. Details, A2.

**Marin Independent Journal**

ember 25, 1991

"January," said Hammer.  | "Plume," will wash away with the first good rain.

**NEWS WATCH**
twatch warns eart attack

from Bob Francisco eam "had y study of commis does meet d by our

**A wristwatch for the heart**

Berkeley physician invents miniature monitor to provide 1-hour warning of cardiac attacks

**La montre qui sauve**

Vous vivez dans l'an-goisse d'une attaque cardiaque? La récente invention d'une montre très spéciale devrait vous tranquilliser. Elle est conçue pour émettre un bip une heure avant que l'infarctus ne s'ins...

By Jayne Garrison
EXAMINER HEALTH WRITER

A Berkeley physician has patented a miniature electrocardiograph monitor the size of a wristwatch that he hopes someday will

This device is an *electrocardiograph monitor invented by a Berkeley sician; it is designed to provide early warning of a heart attack.*

**Herzinfarkt: Frühwarnsystem am Handgelenk** Hauptursache für Infarkttod: Der Patient ist nicht rechtzeitig in der Klinik. Wg. plötzlicher Attacke, keine Hilfe in Sicht. Dr. Kenneth Matsumure aus Berkley, USA, hat ein Infarktfrühwarnsystem erfunden. Eine Sportuhr mit Elektroden, die Änderung der EKG-Signale auffängt. Eine Std. vor Infarkt warnt Piepton; Sofort in die Klinik! Infarktuhr demnächst für ca. 150 Mark im Handel.

Warnung per Piepton: Infarktuhr

Ken also developed his Heart Attack-Alert Wristwatch.™ Ken's watch got global attention with either first or second page news articles, including in countries like Indonesia. In 1999 he received a patent for Computer-Assisted Monitoring of the Body that described both the Egg-Timer™ and Heart Attack-Alert Wristwatch.™[51] But he would never complete the development of either of these products.

In particular, he realized it would be very hard to defend his heart watch device in court because wearers could ignore an alarm and wait too long before going to the emergency room to save their lives. Signed disclaimers would not be an adequate defense. So Ken never developed nor manufactured the watch for sale. Sadly, a needed invention would have to remain unavailable. Shortly after his patent was granted, Apple started producing wristwatches that monitored bodily functions, but their watch does not alert the wearer of a pending heart attack.

He developed one project to purposely by-pass computers. LifeData Card™ [52] is a simple multi-fold card to be carried and easily read. His website Lifedatacard.com describes its use.

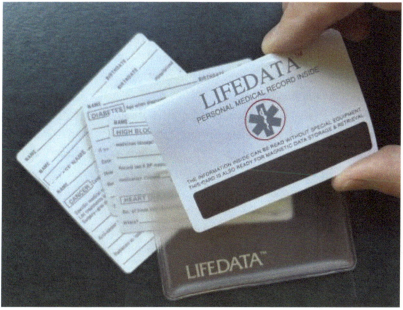

*Available at Lifedatacard.com  see endnote 32*

LifeData Card contains critical information emergency staff can use should the person be alone and not responsive when he or she arrive in ER. The card can be easily updated at the end of any doctor visit, and is meant to be carried with the person at all times. Ken knew as he had worked in the ER at Herrick Hospital that emergency room doctors need to know a patient's medical history in 30 seconds to make life and death decisions. Online records, cell phones, even companions are often not accessible or accurate. Online medical record keeping software has tempered the need for LifeData Cards,™ but is inadequate when patients go to an emergency room not affiliated with the hospital or HMO keeping their record. Ken got outstanding interest in the card from just one senior periodical ad, and his one employee Yvonne Eldridge, who championed the project, was getting lots of inquiries. But Ken didn't carry through with its distribution. He stopped all his projects when Molleen's aunt was diagnosed with breast cancer.

## 19

At Molleen's request, Ken turned his focus towards finding a cure for cancer. Besides solving his family emergency, a cure for cancer would be widely used and produce the funds necessary to defend any of his inventions.

It was 1989 when Miriam was first diagnosed with stage 3 breast cancer. Eleven of her thirteen lymph nodes under her arm were also positive for cancer cells, meaning cancer had already spread. UCSF gave her 2-3 years to live, and her local oncologist in Grants Pass, Oregon advised her to prepare her two children, ages 8 and 12 for her passing. Ken worked with her oncologist who begrudgingly followed his suggestion to use a standard chemo protocol that had achieved 60% long term survival.[53] Even when Miriam experienced extreme nausea, Ken insisted this doctor continue to follow the protocol precisely as it had been done in the study. Miriam reached remission, and for over a decade she was able to raise her children. Then in 2002 cancer returned with a vengeance, this time to the other breast with metastasis spread throughout her liver.[54] Her oncologist could not tell if it was a recurrence of her cancer from 10 years ago, or a new cancer in the other breast.

Sometimes, a recurrence can be determined by comparing the protein on the cells surface with the prior cancer's surface protein. If it is not the same, even though it is the same organ, it can be a new cancer. Even after curing cancer in one organ, cancer can restart in that same organ or in another organ. People who get one cancer are more likely than those who have never had cancer to get a second completely different cancer. Our immune systems do protect us from getting cancer, but some people's immune systems do a better job than others.

The 12 years Miriam was in remission allowed Ken time to concentrate on the idea he had years before to use an antidote to eliminate chemo agent side effects. He hired two UC Berkeley biology undergrads, Christi L. Ober and Scott Storaker, to begin developing his idea into a human therapy. Initially SEF Immuno-Chemo™ used vinblastine as the chemo agent. All in all they tested 21 chemo agents including taxel, methotrexate, cyclophosphamide, and carboplatin. Carboplatin proved superior for killing cancer, and they turned their focus to perfecting its use.

But carboplatin had no known antidote so Ken studied pharmaceutical text books looking for substances whose molecular structure would harmlessly merge and protect good body cells against the poisons of carboplatin. For the better part of ten years he tested possible antidotes by putting them in petri dishes of cultured living cells. If the cells remained healthy, he added carboplatin and watched for the result. When he tested mesna he "discovered" the cultured cells were not harmed when carboplatin was added. There was his start.

During Ken's hearing before the Medical Board, the chemo experts insisted multiple times that mesna was only good for preventing damage to the bladder lining from certain chemo agents. They refused to entertain it could have an "off label" use. Off-label uses for a drug have automatic FDA approval, because the FDA has already determined the drug is safe for human use. As the chemotherapy experts at Ken's trial pointed out mesna was approved for reducing side effects of bladder epithelium caused by the chemo agent ifosfamide. But Ken had deduced that both ifosfamide and carboplatin work in the same way, a mechanism of action called alkylation. Not only did his petri dish experience confirm it was effective, but molecularly it made sense. Mesna is, therefore, also carboplatin's antidote.

Ken and his undergrads made preliminary advances in figuring out how to preferentially deliver an antidote to normal dividing cells. Using the natural greater affinity of normal cells over cancer cells to accept the antidote, and carefully injecting just the right daily antidote dose at specified times before and after the chemo infusion, he was able to achieve enough deliverance differential to reduce chemo side effects, without also protecting the cancer cells to the point where the chemo agent was ineffective.

# 20

A few years later in April 1993 something dramatic happened that brought about the a rapid advance in Ken's work. A colleague from the West Oakland Health Center, Henry Mally, asked how his work was going on FAN-C,™

*FAN-C was SEF Immuno-Chemo's™ original name. It was an acronym for Focused Anti-Neoplastic chemotherapy. Neoplastic means cancer and the therapy focused only on killing the cancer. Ken changed its name about 2010 to Side Effect-Free Chemo™ or SEF Chemo™ pronouncing SEF as "safe" to be more user friendly. It wasn't until after his Medical Board hearing in 2023 that he settled on it's final name SEF Immuno-Chemotherapy.™*

Unaware of the FDA "off-label" rule at the time, Ken told Henry he thought he was almost ready to apply to the FDA for permission to begin clinical trials. He had completed his pre-clinical studies using a MSG-vinblastine combination on large tumors in rats without making the rats sick. He exclaimed it was like seeing a miracle. Not only did the juvenile animals keep eating and growing, after two weeks of weekly treatments the tumor appeared to continue to shrink on its own. At this point he would discontinue treatments. Four weeks later the tumors were indiscernible. He observed the animals for additional years without any recurrence of cancer.

Henry then opened up and told him his cousin, a nurse, and mother to three children ages 7, 10, and 17, was in the hospital dying from metastatic breast cancer. He asked Ken if he might treat her. He didn't expect Ken could cure her or anything like that, but explained she perked up when he told her about Ken's FAN-C™ alternative therapy experiments. She desperately wanted to travel to Sacramento in a few weeks and attend her eldest son's graduation from a prestigious high school academy. Henry told Ken his cousin was willing to take a chance on this new therapy in the hopes it might make her well enough for that trip. Currently, with cancer spread to the liver and lungs she was just too short winded to go.

Ken hesitated because he hadn't submitted a single paper to the FDA. His only contact with the FDA had been a visit that prior Fall with the head of the oncology division in Bethesda, MD. Dr. Ellen Cutler showed intrigue at his idea and he left encouraged. He didn't know at the time FDA approval was not necessary, and evidently, no one knew or thought to tell him otherwise. Vinblastin and its antidote, monosodium glutamate (commonly known as the food additive MSG,) and carboplatin and its antidote mesna were all readily available and already in human use.

That Thursday afternoon, Ken called Henry's cousin Sharon McGee and her oncologist. Her oncologist was a world famous physician who had developed a proprietary procedure of treating advanced cancer patients. His procedure was extremely painful, but at the time proved effective. Patients came from all over the world for his therapy. It was likely, he had a very lucrative practice.

The doctor was enthusiastic and said he had "wards full of patients who could benefit from Ken's approach." He assigned his Executive Assistant to work on getting approval from the University Hospital's Human Subject Experimentation board. Apparently she was very good at getting approval through rapidly. Ken worked all that night producing a 32 page application providing summaries of all pre-clinical laboratory and animal data. He included a cover letter asking if there was any possibility he could be allowed to treat

# FOOD AND DRUG ADMINISTRATION
## OFFICE OF DRUG EVALUATION I
### DIVISION OF ONCOLOGY AND
### PULMONARY DRUG PRODUCTS

Parklawn Building
5600 Fishers Lane
Rockville, MD 20857

## FACSIMILE COVER SHEET

PLEASE DELIVER THE FOLLOWING PAGES TO:

NAME: _____Kenneth Matsumura, M.D._____

LOCATION _Alin Foundation_

510-549-2324

FROM: _____Ellen Cutler_____

Total number of pages, including this cover sheet: __1__

Date: __5-1-02__

If you have any difficulty in receiving this transmission, please contact us at (301) 443-5197 (voice) (301) 443-9284 (FAX)

**THANK YOU**

**COMMENTS:**

As discussed, IND 35,743 has been assigned to you for compassionate treatment of a single patient with FANC-DIRA MSG.

An official letter will be sent by mail and will discuss further responsibilities pertaining to your sponsorship of this IND.

*Ellen*

---

*FDA IND 35,743 compassionate FAN-C trial for 1 patient*

a human patient on a compassionate protocol. He faxed his communication at 5 AM Pacific time, 8 AM Bethesda, MD time. Midday, Dr. Cutler personally called him. She was so impressed by his application and excited by the prospect of a real advance in cancer treatment that she asked directors of her three subdivisions: pharmacology, clinical affairs, and toxicology to take his application home over the weekend.

On Monday three days after submitting his FDA application, Ken received a joint phone call from the three heads of the FDA's subdivisions who had reviewed his work. They asked him a few short questions, which he promptly answered. Then they told him they had decided to approve his application, but as this was a first trial, he must use the lowest dosage of vinblastine on Sharon for the first of her two weekly treatment. Ken had bypassed the months to possibly a year of the usual channels for FDA approval, and was ready to rock and roll.[56]

But things did not go as well at the medical school. After he had submitted his application on Friday, Ken spoke with Sharon's doctor's Executive Assistant several times. He gave her the information she needed to complete her application to the Human Subjects Committee at the hospital. Toward the end of the day, she confided in Ken how upset she was. She had misjudged and made a mistake when Sharon's doctor came into her office. When he asked what she thought about Ken's approach, she enthusiastically said, "Now we won't have to do all those painful procedures!" Immediately, she knew she had misspoken. The doctor's jaw dropped. He said nothing, turned, and left her office. After that he wouldn't return her calls or answer her page. She realized he wasn't going to sponsor the clinical treatment of Sharon McGee. Not only was she upset she was very angry having worked all weekend on this application only to have the doctor bail. Her anger pushed her to take initiative and ask a new oncologist to sponsor Sharon's treatment. He was from MD Anderson, and had just started at the medical school. The new doctor consented right away. He wasn't yet involved in their "specialty" treatment.

The MD Anderson oncologist agreed with Ken that the 0.10 mg per Kg dose of vinblastine, approved for their first treatment by the FDA, would basically be useless. But Ken wasn't about to challenge the FDA, so they agreed to proceed as permitted.

Even while she was continually using oxygen, Sharon was very sick, coughing a lot and very short winded. She was elated the FDA had given approval for Ken to go ahead. Her original oncologist no longer visited, though his office was only a few steps away, and Ken introduced her to the doctor taking over her care.

Sharon was short-winded because cancer had seeded the inside lining of the empty sacs called pleura in which the lungs lie. These sacs reserve the space lungs need to expand and breath deeply. Pleuritic fluid was accumulating in the lung sacs around both her lungs due to these cancer seedlings, and Sharon was limited to unsatisfying frequent small breaths. Every few days doctors would remedy this by inserting a needle into the pleural sac and withdrawing the pleuritic fluid. She could then be comfortable for a few days until fluid built up again.

Ken received the official IND [Investigational New Drug][56] certificate Tuesday. He arrived in Mt. View, California on Thursday ready to administer his first FAN-C™ treatment of MSG and vinblastin into a human. The procedure would take 4 days. Thursday morning before any treatment started, they drew fluid from the lung sacs. The pathology report said the fluid was full of cancer cells visibly dividing with many cells dividing so rapidly that daughter cells were not completely separated before their daughter cells started dividing. There were triplet and quadruplet cells in the pleural fluid.

Ken gave Sharon her first injection of the MSG antidote Thursday evening and again Friday morning. Friday afternoon Sharon received the 0.10 mg per Kg infusion of vinblastine. Saturday, she received an additional injection of the antidote. That afternoon Sharon's lung sacs began to fill with fluid and she became very short-winded. The collaborating doctor placed a needle into Sharon's lung sacs and removed the pleuritic fluid, some of which he sent to the lab. She was comfortable Sunday.

When the pathology report came back on the fluid removed the day after Sharon's treatment, both Ken and the collaborating MD Anderson doctor were shocked. Even using a dose of vinblastine so low it was thought to be useless almost all cancer cells in the pleural

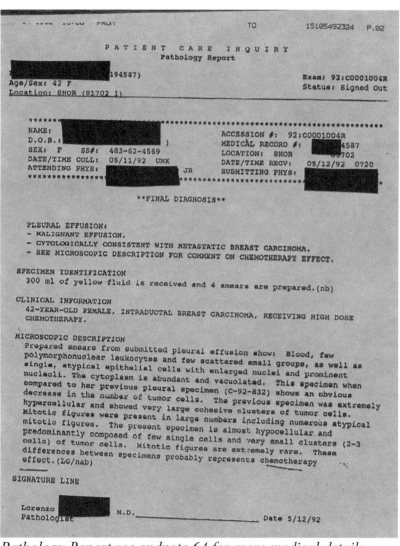

P A T I E N T   C A R E   I N Q U I R Y
Pathology Report

194587)
Age/Sex: 42 F                                    Exam: 92:C0001004R
Location: 8NOR (81702 1)                          Status: Signed Out

NAME:
D.O.B.:                                   ACCESSION #:  92:C0001004R
SEX: F    SS#:  483-62-4569               MEDICAL RECORD #:     4587
DATE/TIME COLL: 05/11/92  UNK             LOCATION: 8NOR         702
ATTENDING PHYS:               JR          DATE/TIME RECV: 05/12/92  0720
                                          SUBMITTING PHYS:

**FINAL DIAGNOSIS**

PLEURAL EFFUSION:
- MALIGNANT EFFUSION.
- CYTOLOGICALLY CONSISTENT WITH METASTATIC BREAST CARCINOMA.
- SEE MICROSCOPIC DESCRIPTION FOR COMMENT ON CHEMOTHERAPY EFFECT.

SPECIMEN IDENTIFICATION
    300 ml of yellow fluid is received and 4 smears are prepared.(nb)

CLINICAL INFORMATION
    42-YEAR-OLD FEMALE, INTRADUCTAL BREAST CARCINOMA, RECEIVING HIGH DOSE
    CHEMOTHERAPY.

MICROSCOPIC DESCRIPTION
    Prepared smears from submitted pleural effusion show:  Blood, few
    polymorphonuclear leukocytes and few scattered small groups, as well as
    single, atypical epithelial cells with enlarged nuclei and prominent
    nucleoli. The cytoplasm is abundant and vacuolated.  This specimen when
    compared to her previous pleural specimen (C-92-832) shows an obvious
    decrease in the number of tumor cells.  The previous specimen was extremely
    hypercellular and showed very large cohesive clusters of tumor cells.
    Mitotic figures were present in large numbers including numerous atypical
    mitotic figures.  The present specimen is almost hypocellular and
    predominantly composed of few single cells and very small clusters (2-3
    cells) of tumor cells.  Mitotic figures are extremely rare.  These
    differences between specimens probably represents chemotherapy
    effect.(LG/nab)

SIGNATURE LINE

    Lorenzo
    Pathologist            M.D._____ Date 5/12/92

*Pathology Report see endnote 64 for more medical details*

fluid had been eradicated!   In addition it appeared the remaining
cancer cells were not dividing.[58] Sharon received a second treatment
starting Thursday of the following week.  She became strong enough
to leave the hospital, travel, and see her son graduate.  Ken told her
to come back as soon as she could.  He speculated that she loved

being out of the hospital and delayed her return until she was again gasping for breath. She was so sick when she did return complications made it impossible to save her.

The FDA trial granted Sharon her humble request to see her son graduate. But her bravery, courage, and love gave cancer research a significant step towards a cure. Her outstanding pathology report results were huge. Ken felt an obligation to speed up the development of SEF Immuno-Chemo.™ He concentrated his energy to focus on saving the more than half million people who die every year from cancer in the U.S. alone.[60]

## 21

Ken considered the sponsor issue of his first FDA trial an outlier, and believed cancer research, pharmaceutical companies, hospitals and oncologists were all dedicated to curing cancer. He wanted to introduce SEF Immuno-Chemo™ to the world. But he didn't have money so he approached the drug companies. His invention would give them their desired outcome and make them lots of money too. Naively, he thought his ask would be a shoo-in.

MCI had given him a $1000 worth of free phone calling anywhere in the world. He drafted a letter to the CEOs of all the pharmaceutical concerns around the world, USA, Europe, Japan, etc. Then he faxed his letter.[61]

He started to get lots of inquiries, many of them from large companies already in cancer care. One by one though, he noticed them losing interest. It was puzzling, until one executive of a large European company explained in confidence to Ken that as drug companies are mostly public concerns everything they do has to be towards maximizing profits for their share holders. They had to measure Ken's therapy, not for its purpose or effectiveness, but against products that could make continuous money. Their products were designed to extend the lives of cancer patients. When one product stops working the drug company would have a second product to further extend life, then a third, and so on. If a product completely cures a cancer victim that patient is no longer a customer,

<u>and there would be no more sales.</u> He complimented Ken by saying SEF Chemo™ was a wonderful breakthrough, but as a money-maker, a poor product. It was a moment of reality. Ken's naivety dropped away. There would be no help.

Contrary to their promising ads, contrary to accepting billions of dollars in donations, contrary to the intention cited as the reason we gave billions of our tax dollars to the recent "Moonshot" funding,[62] the medical world was in 2003 and remains today not interested in embracing a technology that would kill their golden goose. Ken's marketing efforts to introduce SEF Chemo™ and assure people of its efficacy are summarily negated by the very industry he cherished. SEF Immuno-Chemo™ remains obscure, cancer's cure unrealized, and a pipeline of medical advances, which SEF's™ funds could have released, unbirthed.

New York Times columnist David Brooks said, "It is better to trust people than not to." Extrapolating on his thought, I feel trust fuels optimism and fortifies courage. It is one of the foundational blocks of happiness. Ken accepted his disappointment and vowed to go on. He would proceed alone.

## 22

To give the drug companies the benefit of the doubt I don't think they minded eliminating the side effects of their chemo drugs. That would have been a big selling point. They just didn't want to promote something that had even limited data showing tumors in rats or mice dissolving.

Ken wondered how his antidote was making chemotherapy more effective too. For most of a year he studied, trying to understand what seemed to be a miracle. It wasn't until he remembered a lecture in one of his medical school physiology classes that he realized, besides guarding our bodies against bacterial infections, the white blood neutrophils of our immune system also seek out sick, injured, and aged cells. Once the neutrophils find these cells they use a divine [extremely good] system to phagocytize [dissolve] them.[63] Apparently, the antidote in SEF Immuno-Chemo™

was keeping neutrophil cells alive and protecting the immune system that conventional chemotherapy destroys. It appeared that after a SEF Immuno-Chemo™ treatment a patient's immune system was still healthy, and the industrious neutrophils could continue their grand work.

The unplanned continued eradication of cancer after a SEF Chemo™ treatment made Ken recognize chemo agents are extremely limited in their ability to kill cancer cells. To cure cancer you need to kill a lot more cancer cells with each treatment than chemo agents can kill alone. But with the help of each patient's champion neutrophils the race between the patient and their cancer could now be consistently won for the patient. SEF Chemo™ wasn't curing cancer, but SEF Immuno-Chemo™ was.

# 23

When Molleen's Aunt Miriam, came out of remission in 2002, she had cancer in both breasts, in more lymph nodes and in her liver. Ken had successfully tested vinblastine with its MSG antidote on another human. So he began treatment on Miriam. She tolerated it without many, if any, side effects. However, after a year, her cancer had continued to spread and was worse. He realized she needed something more powerful. He was working with her oncologist who agreed to try drugs in the vinca series of cancer drugs, all similar to vinblastine. This family of drugs is usually used in combination with other chemo drugs, which Ken did not have antidotes for. Plus, no drugs in the vinca series are as powerful as carboplatin. Carboplatin is often used alone, because it effectively kills more types of cancer, even cells that try to transform themselves to be resistant to the chemo agent. With most drugs, including vinca drugs, if the cancer starts to change, you have to change the drug. Since carboplatin and its antidote mesna were both already approved as safe by the FDA, Ken now knew he was free to employ them for "off-label" use. Late in 2002 Miriam's results were still not improving. Her liver had become three times larger than normal.

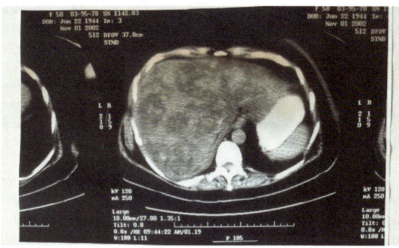

*Liver CT Scan before SEF treatments*

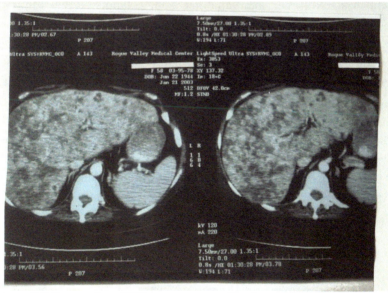

*Liver CT Scan after SEF treatments. Each cancer lesion is outlined because cancer turned to water.*

Ken had completed animal tests with carboplatin and mesna in November, and they showed promising results. So in the last week of December he started Miriam on an alternating weekly protocol.

He used low dose AUC 2 carboplatin the first week then low dose gemcitabine at 300 mg per $M^2$ the second week. This he repeated over six weeks. A few days after her third cycle Miriam's liver enzymes went way up. Her bile pigment, called bilirubin, was more than 10 times normal. People look jaundiced when it is twice normal. Her oncologist ordered another CT scan. The scan confirmed positive results. Her liver metastasis had completely liquified.[65]

Ken was back in Berkeley where he was receiving Miriam's test results. He saw her CT scan, the radiologist comments, and her blood tests. Her blood tests showed her bilirubin falling. Already it had changed from 10 to 9 mg %. He believed her cancer was finally responding. The treatment had been a success.

But there was discord in Grants Pass. His presence was needed to reassure them. He traveled to Oregon joining his wife, Molleen, who was with her aunt and her aunt's family. But Miriam's oncologist had made her own interpretation of the x-rays. Miriam was already in hospice and on a morphine drip for pain. So her oncologists told Miriam and her family that Miriam's liver was coming apart and death was imminent. Ken talked with Miriam, but on morphine she would go along with anything. He tried to reason with her oncologist, but was over-ruled. The oncologist let the morphine drip continue, and Miriam passed away a few days later from morphine overdose. After her own mother's early death Molleen's aunt had become her surrogate mother. Now, heartbroken, Molleen, stayed in Oregon to bury her beloved aunt.

## 24

Ken excitedly contacted the MD Anderson oncologist who collaborated with him when treating Sharon McGee and was now in private practice in Texas. But his excitement was met with disdain and hostility, and he was told to never call again.

It pains me to hear my sweet husband endured such rejection. Marketing for cancer patients is intense. Ken's google ads are no match for the big pharmaceutical companies and hospitals who have enough money to sponsor their ads at the top of the first search page. Nor does Ken have the money to compete with their slick TV ads that promise so much before adding a list of side effects in a flurry of tachylalia. Ken's name is not displayed on any large and impressive buildings like the high-rise "Stanford Cancer Center" looming over the highway 87 / 17 exchange in San Jose, California.

Four years ago a good friend's boyfriend was diagnosed with lung cancer. Even though Ken had prior success putting three lung cancer patients into long term remission, the most recent now for over six years, my friend told me her boyfriend preferred to go to a renown cancer hospital in Texas. There he paid them $37,000 for four days of their expert analysis. With prescription in hand he returned to Kaiser in California where he was a Medicare Advantage member. Kaiser was already familiar with the therapy and willingly followed the recommendation. His response was minimal. Another friend of my same friend, when diagnosed with lung cancer decided to go to a well advertised cancer center on the San Francisco Bay Area peninsula. At her initial appointment her companion reported they told her "she could live another 5 years if they treated her." Five years must have sounded pretty good to a ninety-year-old. I understand she took their advice, but died shortly after completing their therapy. Treatment did not give her what she'd hoped for, but, it was a complete advertising success for the cancer center.

## 25

Cancer care has become a billions of dollars business.[67] The abuse that Ken foresaw when he worked at West Oakland Health Clinic in 1965 has manifested. Cancer research and treatments lead that abuse.[66] Oncologists themselves make nearly twice the amount of money pediatricians make.[68] And pediatricians have to get up at all hours of the night to take care of their young patients.

While it's true drug companies make drugs for all types of ailments, cancer research that produces drugs for both chemotherapy and now immune therapy top the list of money makers.[69] The latest FDA approved cancer care drugs are the new immune therapy drugs.

They're also big players in the government funded "Moonshot" 2016 directive to cure cancer.[70] Immune therapies typically starts at a mere $30 thousand per treatment before price blasting into the stratosphere.[71] Although they regularly cite R&D expenses as the reason for the exorbitant price, a recent JAMA Network Open publication found no connection between what is spent on research and development for a drug and the drug's retail value.[72] In addition, a lot of R&D is funded through generous donations and tax dollars. So it's an expense that has its own source of financing. Between 2016 and 2020 cancer research global funding was 24.5 billion with the U.S. contributing 57.3% of that.[73] Unfortunately, only a quarter of that funding is slated to improve radiotherapy and cancer surgery – two procedures regularly offered to cancer patients.[74] Though big pharmaceutical companies "must" still beg for money, kudos to the top 20 in the U.S. who have, somehow, managed to eek-out billions of dollars in profits.[75]

As of August 2024 the FDA has approved numerous new immune therapies drugs.[76] I went down an internet rabbit hole on Cancer Research Institute's (CRI) website. I didn't cherry pick. Tecelra® was listed first. It is a CAR T-based immune therapy, their newest marvel, and it targets one cancer type, synovial sarcoma. After a clinical trial involving 44 patients the FDA approved Tecelra® because it showed "remarkable" efficacy.[77]

Response, remission and cure are meaningful words to express positive results in cancer care. But they're often used by doctors and advertisers and end up confusing hopeful people, by implying possibilities that may not be true. Response means after receiving a treatment a patient's cancer changes for the better. It grows slower or shrinks in size. It hasn't gone away. Remission means the conventional tests for cancer cannot detect cancer. But cancer can and may still be present. Once a patient is said to be in remission, cancer treatment is suspended, until cancer is again detected with a followup test. Remission is the first goal. Cure means a patient has remained in remission for 5 preferably 10 years, and of course, cure is the patient's real goal.

I would guess the FDA's "remarkable" descriptor for 43.2% of the 44 trial patients meant 19 got a response. I doubt it meant the patients went into remission or were cured. No mention was made of what happened to the other 26 people. I would've hoped they'd have used the correct word, "remission," if indeed 43.2% achieved it. Remission is something to brag about, and the word is generally understood. Since Tecelra® is a "one time solves it" treatment,[78] if it indeed was only response, and not remission, the FDA might have wanted to frame the result, they were about to approve, to sound, well — more — remarkable.

Why would the FDA approve a one time treatment therapy that wasn't even stopping cancer with it's one treatment? Possibly the reason, not found on the CRI's website was Tecelra's® $727,000 price tag.[79] Is the FDA really looking out for us?

Also, not included, on the CRI website, were the side effects of Tecelra.®[80] So using Google, I queried "side effects of Tecelra.®" Hmm, maybe the FDA should have done that! Seems 20% **or more** patients experience nausea, vomiting, tiredness, constipation, fever (100.4°F/38°C or higher), infection, abdominal pain, difficulty breathing, decreased appetite, diarrhea, low blood pressure, back pain, fast heart rate, chest pain, general body swelling, low white blood cells, low red blood cells, and low platelets. Those were the lucky ones! Because with this "remarkable" medicine, 5% **or more** of the patients get cytokine release syndrome and pleural effusion, which are fatal side effects where abnormal fluid accumulates within the thin space surrounding the lungs.[81]

Between 2013 and 2017 Ken partnered with Dr. Akbar Khan. With Ken's daily oversight and counseling Dr. Khan offered SEF Immuno-Chemo™ at his Medicore Clinic in Toronto, Canada. He published each individual's SEF™ results on the clinic's website. The average response rate for the 76 patients who received SEF Immuno-Chemo during the three years Dr. Khan offered SEF™ was 87%,[82] twice the response rate of the "remarkable" Tecelra.® Estimating Khan's patients each received an average of 8 treatments at $5 thousand each, SEF's™ cost was .006 of Tecelra's.® The pharmaceutical companies who jockeyed for the authority to inform

Vice President Biden were careful not to invite Ken and his FDA approved Side Effect Free Immuno-Chemo™ aboard the Moonshot.

## 26

Cancer research is constantly soliciting for greater funding. But maximizing dollars doesn't stop there. Pharmaceutical companies have created many more schemes. A few tricks include extending patents by tweaking an existing drug so they can patent it as a brand-new drug,[83] merge with another drug company to avoid price competition,[84] and sell their old drugs to other pharmaceutical companies, so those companies can double or triple the price.[85]

I recently needed to buy some iodine to make a simple douche. Ken stood next to me in the CVS line. While we waited we both guessed what the unmarked bottle would cost based on our estimate of inflation. I said $7; he said $6. It rang as $27.99. I face-planted on the cashier's COVID shield, paid, and staggered out of the store. At home, before opening the new bottle, I rechecked my medicine drawer. There in the very back, shining like a beacon of joy, was an old bottle of precious iodine. Its faded sticker read $6.62. I returned the new purchase, and hope to never-ever have to buy iodine again.

But my iodine was no big deal compared to the experimental prescriptions for new subpar drugs. 8.1 billion was spent in 2022 alone on advertising to introduce and boost demand for these new drugs. Ads to tantalizes the public with magic cures while down playing the many side effects add to the cost of all drugs. During the six years of the study, "Only about one in four of these heavily advertised drugs had high therapeutic value. Between 2015-21 pharmaceutical companies spent an estimated $15.9 billion advertising 73 drugs a quarter of which showed no advantage over the drugs they purported to replace"[86] Drug-sales people leave samples of new drugs with doctors in the hopes of enticing them to switch from the tried and true medicines they've come to rely on. Unwittingly, doctors oblige the drug companies by passing out these free samples to many patients so they can save money on their initial prescription costs. Of course, some just take the pharmaceutical sales person's spiel and start prescribing. A close friend of mine has Crohns. Unfortunately, she's been in and out of hospitals for over 20 years. After one visit she remarked to Ken that they finally gave her a wonderful new medication that really worked. With 45 years as an internist, Ken told her it was hardly new. He said balsalazide is a common medicine that's been in use for many years to relieve digestive problems.

## 27

There is, within the pharmaceutical distribution chain, a stealth player. Pharmacy Benefit Managers are contracted to negotiate prices between drug manufacturers, insurance companies, employers, pharmacies, and Medicare Part D for drugs. PBM are often pharmacists with a background in insurance, though some only have a bachelor's degree in science.[87] This symbiotic relationship between PBMs and drug companies dictates how PBMs weigh their choices.

PBMs make the final coverage decisions for drugs and assign codes to each. All insurance claims must reference an appropriate billing code to receive reimbursement. PBMs also decide how much of this cost is passed on to patients. Criteria authored by the National Association of Insurance Commissioners [NAIC] states, "within the generally accepted standards of medical care in the community."[88] It appears to be the only excuse I see as a reason not to create billing codes for SEF Immuno-Chemo.™ By using the non-specific words, "generally," "accepted," "standards," and "community," it is difficult to know precisely what Ken needs to do to change his standing. The "community" that is deciding and accepting the standards must be comprised of oncologists, hospitals, pharmaceutical companies including their PBM contractors, and insurance executives. It can't be referring to the general public. Because without insurance coverage SEF Immuno-Chemo™ is out of reach for most of that "community."

As contractors, the PBM's fees and incentives are conveniently based on a share of the total cost for the medicines they negotiate.

PBMs "account for 42% of every dollar spent on brand medicines in the commercial market,"[89] So they're not likely approve insurance payments for a competitor whose drugs are less expensive, and especially, for one whose product is not designed to gain profit from returning customers. PBMs can put the kibosh on all threats to the status quo. They may well be where the buck stops for SEF Immuno-Chemo.™

Insurance company executives, hospitals and oncologists, pharmaceutical companies and PBMs protect their turf, and claim they do it all for the public good. Unable to understand the tangled rhetoric of insurance and pharmaceutical companies, we accept the decisions and opinions they use to increase co-pays, deductibles, and premiums, while we watch our national debt rise and our personal expenses increase. Healthy people are, therefore, not exempt from the high cost of health care.

Many of Ken's SEF™ patients and the many more who applied to be treated attempted to get insurance coverage. Ken composed an informational letter and gave it to each of them to include with their request.[90] In it he explained SEF Immuno-Chemo™ in detail, gave results, and compared it to conventional chemotherapy and immune therapy. Each SEF Immuno-Chemo™ treatment cost between $4 and $6 thousand, and patients, who were not advanced beyond stage 3, were typically spending around 50-80 thousand dollars to reach remission. It was a price cheaper than any cancer therapy in the world. In his letter Ken also spoke of the human toll. He included that many of the terminal cancer sufferers who came to him had been dismissed as hopeless by their oncologists. He gave proof that SEF Immuno-Chemo™ had or could turn their cancer around, and remission was possible. But no amount of proof, price, or pleading produced billing codes to cover the cost for SEF Immuno-Chemo.™ "Denied" was always the answer. Those without financial means quietly stopped corresponding with Ken or quit SEF™ before they were through to bravely face the outcome of their disease.

SEF Immuno-Chemo™ is not a trial drug. Since 2003 it has been administered and sold commercially to the few patients who could afford it. For those few, it achieved responses, remissions, and cures even when their cancers were considered hopeless. SEF Immuno-Chemo™ satisfies NAIC's[91] definition of an insurable medically necessary treatment which "provided for the diagnosis, treatment, cure, or relief of a health condition, illness, injury, or disease...." It is not "experimental, investigational, or used for cosmetic purposes." But as of today, SEF Immuno-Chemo™ is still not covered by insurance.

Here's an example of what we're getting for our hard earned money with conventional chemotherapy. In 2015 a man came to Ken after being treated with conventional cancer therapy for 7 years. He had  aggressive prostate cancer. His was their success story because he had outlived the life expectancy for aggressive prostate cancer.[91] He was on Medicare, which pays 80%, and he also had a supplemental insurance through AT&T his former employer that paid the remainder. He gave Ken a raft of bills showing "we" had paid over 3 million for his care. The sterling result of our investment was that cancer had spread all over his body, and his life was miserable because of his pain. Yes, he had outlived the statistics, but he didn't go through all that therapy just to outlive someone's table of numbers. Now his doctors admitted they couldn't cure him, something they did know or should have known all along. So he refused hospice care and started to look around for alternatives. By the time he found Berkeley-Institute and SEF Immuno-Chemo,™ Ken couldn't give him what he wanted. He had suffered with cancer too long, and too many of his organs had been compromised beyond their ability to recover. However, he improved dramatically with SEF.™ After only a month he was going out to eat at restaurants with his family, and his wife said he was better than he had been in all his prior years of treatment. He ate, he sang, and played his guitar (they were all musicians.) He laughed and he loved. A year after his death, his son, who had delayed his marriage while the family concentrated on the father's illness, invited us to his beautiful outdoor wedding. They still mourned the loss of their honored patriarch. He will never be forgotten. But they will always be grateful to Ken for bringing happiness back into their last few months together.

71

Unless people have had prior experience with cancer, they usually default to getting their treatments where insurance will cover them. Americans especially experience sticker shock when they find out each SEF Immuno-Chemo™ treatment costs thousands of dollars. But if they considered what insurance and Medicare were paying for conventional cancer treatments, costs that are shared by everyone, they would understand better why our national debt is constantly rising and realize SEF Immuno-Chemo™ is our nation's most cost-effective option.

## 28

Until the Inflation Reduction Act (IRA)[92] was enacted, the U.S. unlike other nations let drug and biologic manufacturers set whatever prices they wanted. Fortunately, on August 16, 2022, President Biden signed IRA into law. Finally, we have a law that gives us what was needed since Medicare's inception 60 years ago, a seat at the healthcare negotiating table. I believe the Inflation Reduction Act is poorly named because while doing many good things it doesn't control inflation or prevent corporations from raising their prices. Regardless of the poor name, the Inflation Reduction Act is one of the largest investments in the American economy, energy security, and climate remediation in our nation's history. It makes Medicare stronger for current and future enrollees. It makes healthcare more accessible, equitable, and affordable by lowering what Medicare spends for prescription drugs and by limiting increases in prices. Drug price negotiation will begin with just 10 drugs and will start to be felt in 2026. Meanwhile, a $2,000 cap will help limit drug costs for 65 million people on Medicare in the U.S.[93] If you are not on Medicare, know that the prices it sets are also used by insurance companies who offer insurance coverage for all ages.[94]

The Inflation Reduction Act was a phenomenal achievement for our government officials who faced off against the healthcare industry. They weren't "speaking truth to power." Our President earns $400,000 a year.[95] They were "speaking truth to people making 100 times and more what they make." We're lucky healthcare representatives even showed up to talk. Sustained rigorous effort by American citizens is needed if we don't want the Inflation Reduction Act to be the sole lifeline we get to control healthcare costs. Because without continuing to improve healthcare through mediation the American dream of raising a family and aging gracefully will become the American mirage.

*In endnote [96] I have listed the state and federal bills pending legislative action to expose and transform what PBMs do. Please look at them, and if you approve, call your representatives to ask them to push these bills along. There is no bigger or better lobby than thousands of citizens calling their representative with specific requests for them to co-author, vote for, or introduce a particular bill.*

# 29

Ken's Medical Licensing Board hearing in August of 2023 was not for malpractice. It was a "complaint investigation" consisting of three complaints. One made by an oncologist and one made by a hospitalist-physician[97] who had no cancer treatment training. They represented families of patients who were still within the statue of limitation to sue for malpractice, but were not interested in doing so. The third complaint was by the ex-husband of one of Ken's patients. His wife had leaned upon him to pay for her SEF™ treatment, after their divorce had financially destroyed her. Over the 45 years that Ken saw thousands of patients during office visits and hospital admissions, he maintained a perfect record. He had never received any complaint by the doctors he had worked with. Nor had he ever been accused of malpractice by patients who felt mistreated.[98]

In the last few years we've heard more and more stories of cancer patients avoiding ordinary oncologists. Many of the patients who came to Ken for SEF Immuno-Chemo™ were referred by his prior patients or people who'd heard good things about him. Even though cancer diagnoses and its steady supply of patients remains high, oncologists began to notice more people were questioning their methods and asking for alternatives. Initially the board dismissed some of the complaints from oncologists, but finally decided to adjudicate two of them when they received a complaint from the ex-husband. I have included in the endnotes the order by Judge Juliet E. Cox.[3] It is public record. But Ken's [respondent] defense is part of a closed trial transcript and contains HIPPA information about the three patients represented. It is not available for the public to read. Needless to say I have tried to present his side.

The first complaint was instigated by the hospitalist-physician for Patient One, a 67 year old attorney from Arizona. Not wanting the toxicity of ordinary chemo, she let her breast cancer progress while she searched for alternatives. By the time she came to Ken in 2018 it had metastasized into her liver and lymph nodes. In 2018 Ken was still trying to avoid terribly advanced cases and told her so. She said, she understood she was too advanced, but asked to be treated on a "compassionate" basis anyway. She also asked for a $2 thousand per treatment discount. I meeean – at what point does a request for "compassion" slip into just asking to "take advantage of someone being nice,"... but he gave it to her, even though he ended up spending an inordinate amount of time tending to her needs because of her advanced stage and forceful personality.

Ken decided to treat her using a lower dose carboplatin, so as not to create too much cancer carnage and give her system time to heal after each treatment. He was impressed at how well she tolerated her SEF™ treatments. Initially she was going to move closer to Berkeley, but decided against it because she was still working at her law office in Arizona and her clients needed her there. As she was feeling strong, she and her husband began to drive between home and Berkeley for her bi-weekly SEF™ treatments. Ken worried this would ultimately deplete her energy, and found air flights with pilots donating their labor and a plane to shuttle medical patients to and from their medical appointments.

After ten months, the patient's law partner gave notice. Consequently, Patient One felt she could no longer come to the Bay Area at all. She chose to tend to her clients, rather than continue her self care. Both she and her husband said her malignant lymph nodes,

74

those under hers arm and in her neck were disappearing. Although Ken told her she needed another three months of treatment, she decided she no longer needed SEF.™ He didn't argue. Interestingly a month later, she felt well enough to take a long flight to the East Coast. While flying, she apparently didn't move her legs much and developed a blood clot in her calf. Soon more clots developed in her lungs. A busy emergency room doctor in Arizona saw her cancer diagnosis, and construed that the pain caused from her lung clots must be pain from cancer. The doctor loaded her with huge doses of morphine and Oxycontin and created an addict. Patient One eventually returned to the Bay Area where she was admitted to Sutter Hospital in Oakland. There her single demand was for more morphine. Her husband was beside himself and helpless to solve her addiction. A hospitalist, with virtually no experience in cancer therapy, intervened. She didn't realize image tests after immune cancer therapy show abnormal outlines of organs. It's not until the immune cells complete their work that tumors look smaller or disappear. She misread Patient One's image scan, and told the patient's husband his wife was dying "from cancer." This was very upsetting as the husband had had every confidence in Ken's SEF Immuno-Chemotherapy.™ The disheartened husband allowed the doctor to place his wife in hospice where she could get all the drugs she wanted before dying.

Ken submitted 26 pages of notes describing in detail how SEF Immuno-Chemo™ was eradicating Patient One's cancer. Yet the pages of his notes were not considered when determining the verdict. Using lack of record keeping as one of their primary reasons to revoke his license, the order reiterated the medical board's claim that Ken wasn't keeping medical records for Patient One. Possibly, justice is so blind, Ken should have submitted them in braille.

The second complaint was made by an oncologist who worked at the same HMO (Health Maintenance Organization,) where Patient Two worked as a coronary care nurse. Patient Two had already endured several years of their toxic chemotherapy. When her colon cancer continued to get worse and worse, she decided she needed to try something else. When she approached Dr. Matsumura she was already so advanced and in such poor condition that Ken discouraged her from starting SEF.™ She understood, but liked the concept of his therapy and believed his results. She contested saying she had no other option, and she was not ready to give up. Ken changed his mind.

Even though it was now obvious more of the HMO's treatments would be useless, they refused to cooperate with their employee-member's choice to go out-of-network. They didn't want to spend more money. As a nurse she should have appreciated the HMO's best efforts and graciously accepted their unavoidable results? Instead, while she was receiving SEF™ treatments they routinely refused to run blood tests or give her simple additional procedures that would have drastically stabilized her condition and made her more comfortable. Finally, without regular supportive procedures, she died. When the HMO's oncologist complained to the Medical Board, the nurse's husband was so incensed he refused to cooperate and would not sign permission to release her medical record. This forced the Medical Board to go to a judge and get a subpoena[98] for its release.

*NOTE: Whether a HMO member is treated or not, HMOs are self-insured medical facilities. They receive their support monthly through member premiums and Medicare payments. Any treatment that the HMO has to undertake is an unwelcome cost. Senator Elizabeth Warren has complained that the relentless monthly cost of HMOs is what is bankrupting Medicare.*[99]

The third complaint was made by Patient Three's ex-husband whom she had leaned upon after their divorce to pay for her SEF Immuno-Chemo™ treatment. He did pay, but Ken's medical note said that when the patient brought her ex with her to treatment, his only question was "how soon can she be over with this therapy." The medical board and Judge Cox were seemingly unaware of Patient Three's personal financial issues and that in fact the husband, who was making the complaint, was divorced from the patient.

Patient Three had asked Ken for a discount and he had lowered her treatment cost from $6,000 to $4,200 per treatment. Ken was honest with them and told them SEF™ treatment would take longer and be more expensive because her oncologist had continued treating her despite her cancer getting progressively worse. Due to financial problems Patient Three decided on her own to quit all therapies, including SEF Immuno-Chemo,™ and left to live with her daughter in Oregon before she had any chance of reaching remission.

At the time of Patient Three's enrollment the cost for other SEF Immuno-Chemo™ patients was $6,000. Regardless of whether or not Ken gave a patient a discount he tested the chemo agent for potency. Chemo agent mass potency testing done by pharmaceutical companies cost between $2-3 hundred thousand dollars. Hospital oncologists don't routinely retest the agents even though transporting the medicines is not controlled by the FDA regulations. Although traditional oncological medicines typically cost between $10,000 to $150,000, and even $727,000 per treatment, the medical board accused Ken of financially abusing his patients by adding in an additional cost of $2 thousand to cover testing of the chemo agent's potency.

Judge Juliet E. Cox's order recommending Ken's license be revoked was grueling. She must have felt quite smug "solving our health care crisis" by picking on one man rather than appraising and evaluating the shortcomings of our entire medical industry. She dismissed the opinion of the FDA's three oncology division department heads who saw Ken's extensive cancer research and experience qualified him as principle investigator for SEF Immuno-Chemo's™ clinical trial in 1991.[135] She made countless references to Ken not following the "standard of care" set by a community of adversaries who will likely lose business if Ken is allowed to succeed. She claimed Ken's charges created a greater hardship for his patients while forgetting about the billions of dollars we all pay to keep our medical institutions alive. She ignored his copious notes (OMG, there are so many) on his procedures and patient interaction. Rather than admit he invented something new that would upend the cancer care ruse, she called him a delusional liar. Lastly, her greatest feat, she "protected public safety" by snatching the cancer industry's failure from the jaws of success.

# 30

The cancer care industry sits on a foundation of insurance coverage. If SEF Immuno-Chemo™ were the preferred therapy, a lot of that industry would be unnecessary. There would be no need to concoct the next drug for cancer "management," and no need for medical students to spend additional years in medical school to learn the cornucopia of chemo agents that modulate cancer treatment. With two to three years of supervised training SEF Immuno-Chemo™ can be administered by nurses and general practitioners.

People wouldn't hesitate to be diagnosed or seek cancer treatment because it wouldn't be toxic or life altering. Today, due to the side effects of conventional treatment, oncologists often use suppressant medicines to slow cancer growth. These medicines allow a cancer victim to continue a normal life uninterrupted by the misery of treatment for as long as possible. But suppressants are not a path to remission, and ultimately cancer will kill you.

Patients could start SEF™ treatments long before the disease became life threatening. Early detection and treatment saves time and money. When patients have come to Ken while cancer is still in stage 1 or 2, that is when it has not spread beyond the originating organ, even if it's in a vital organ, SEF™ has often been able to put them in long term remission with 8 infusions given 2 weeks apart over 4 months. These people were able to continue working while in treatment. If cancer had spread to lymph nodes, stage 3, or metastasized in other organs, even vital organs, stage 4, it is still treatable and remission possible with SEF,™ but remission will take longer.

Each cycle of treatment is 3 to 4 days. One day for a chemo agent infusion typically taking less than an hour, and time for a shot of antidote on the day before and one to two days after, depending on the amount of carboplatin infused. <u>Our national cost for health care</u>

would drop through the floor because cancer would be a completely outpatient treatable disease without need for hospitalization.

# 31

Lack of insurance coverage didn't just create problems for people without the means to pay. It kept enrollment so low it was impossible for Ken to expand. At its peak he had only four clinics and five providers available to administer SEF Immuno-Chemo™— not nearly enough to generate the revenue needed to open more clinics in convenient locations. So patients who could afford the treatments had to also be able to afford and endure the inconvenience, and ofttimes boredom, of living away from home, family, and job. _

Ken has tried to share, announce, and advertise his therapy. But he didn't have the money to expand services when the pharmaceutical companies were not interested. He knew if he persisted and succeeded in reaching the millions of cancer sufferers across the United States or further, his limited size would prevent him from helping them. For many years he concentrated his effort only on those with advanced cancer, who he thought were still treatable with SEF.™ He did this to avoid agitating conventional therapy providers. His ads purposely did not try to interest patients who could succeed with conventional chemotherapy. Only patients who were totally adverse to toxicity of conventional chemotherapy or people who had watched a love one die with cancer treatment searched hard enough to find him.

# 32

In neonatal ICUs, "lack of the will to live" is often cited as the cause of death. I remember reading a story about premature twins. They were both small, but one was pretty healthy and doing OK. At the time of the story it was customary to separate twins at birth into different incubators. The smaller one was struggling. It became obvious she wasn't going to make it. The astute mother insisted they be put together in the same incubator. The nurse placed them close, and the bigger twin put her arm over her sister's little shoulders. The smaller child immediately responded to her sister's tender loving care, and they both survived.[32]

SEF Immuno-Chemo™ has a secret ingredient. Ken can't prescribe it, can't document it, can't order it, didn't discover it or invent it. But without it, there is a much greater chance the patient will die from cancer regardless of the therapy they choose. That secret ingredient is TLC, tender loving care.

When Ken and I talk about his patients he always includes family dynamics. Who came with them to their first appointment? Is everyone in favor of going "out of plan" and using their own money to pay? While their loved one is in therapy, are they willing to drive their family member to appointments or relocate? Can they put their needs on-hold to let their family member concentrate on getting better? Over the course of several years we've observed some amazing answers to these questions.

Money is where the family support system seems to be most evident. Recently a thirty year old patient asked her parents to pay for her SEF™ therapy. Even though SEF™ had data showing lots of prior successes, the parents only agreed if she would first submit to a free trial that as yet had no proven success. You see, the medicine is FREE, when you're the lab rat. After her trial treatments ended, her cancer had spread, and the parents consented to pay for SEF Immuno-Chemo.™ She survived, but had to get more treatments to reach remission then she would have, had she foregone the trial and started SEF™ right away.

Positive support and positive companionship is vital. There is a physiological reaction to stress. The adrenal gland's stress hormone cortisone increases when a person is under stress and can damage or kill neutrophils regardless of whether or not you have cancer. Even though neutrophils are not destroyed during a SEF Immuno-Chemo™ treatment, stressed patients experience poorer response because their neutrophils aren't as effective at dissolving the dead and dying cancer cells. Blood test results due to stress can also cause treatments delays, and delay is cancer's friend because cancer grows relentlessly. More cancer means remission takes longer to reach and will be more expensive. Usually more expense means more stress. Commitment, patience, and courage for both family and patient are necessary.

There is no insurance billing code for emotional support. That's obvious from the horror stories patients have told us about the lack of personal attention that their former oncologists had given them. They felt a lack of privacy during a chemo infusion and a lack of clear information about the outcome they could expect from the toxic process. I used to work in the IT department of a HMO. While fixing a doctor's computer, I overheard a phone call she made to a patient. She said, "You're seeing double because there's something inside at the top of your nose, and it's growing. It'll have to grow back before you get better. I'm referring you to the oncology department. They will call you to setup an appointment." I could tell the patient was confused. The doctor repeated louder, "It just needs to grow back!" Then she got off and mumbled, "Too bad, nice girl, only 26." It seemed to me an in-person appointment to break that kind of news might be warranted. But, like I said, no code.

On another occasion a co-worker of mine was diagnosed with cancer. Geri was hands-down the sweetest person you'd ever meet. She never complained about the people, work, pay, or the grueling overtime hours. She was tough, a mother of four, and a doting wife. She was also totally dedicated to her job, "a real company man." But after she met with her oncologist, she told me, "She [who was both her oncologist and the hospital CEO] didn't sound hopeful nor concerned. More indifferent than anything else. And I always gave her such good service. I always made her computer issues my top priority. She was never down or inconvenienced. I made sure everything was just how she wanted it."

My personal experience with the head of the oncology department at the same HMO didn't involve a cancer diagnosis, but certainly exposed an unhappy professional. I was managing a new computer operating system roll-out and we were rebuilding everyone's computers. I created a backup script to collect each doctor's files from all their applications. Both my managers approved the program. We proceeded. I must have stopped at the oncologist's office five times to ask if he knew of anything else he had on his computer. He was good. After the rebuild he called. Furious. He was missing his contacts. I was empathetic. To lose your contacts is a terrible thing. I totally agreed. But he had been using a non-sanctioned email program that he didn't tell me about. No one else in the hospital used that program. He raved, "Tell me who's in charge of this roll-out. Because I'm going to come and beat their head in with a baseball bat." I said, "I am." That ended our phone call, but not the incident. He took it to the head of the hospital. My manager presented my documentation, including the phone call transcript. I guess they resolved it. I was not reprimanded, and I never spoke with that doctor again.

It's certainly understandable oncologists might be in a bad mood. They must get tired of seeing their patients suffer and die. What a thankless job. I wonder if they ever question whether the exorbitant money they make and extra years of education are worth it. In 1969 Kubler Ross wrote the book *On Death and Dying.* Her story gave the nurses' point of view during cancer care. It is the nurses who are left, after the doctor quits coming. Nurses are the ones who have to see the pleading looks. They stay and explain to the distraught, frustrated and tired family members that nothing else can be done. They sympathize. They are gentle. They arrange for hospice.

Ken loves life. He won't let anything die. He waters the weeds and won't pull any. It drives me nuts. His 45 year old Koi fish, Minoru, recently had hundreds of babies, and the pond will soon be packed. He's looking for homes for them. His love of life drives him, and underpins his medical motivation.

The doctor, Ken worked with longest, is a board certified oncologist and surgeon. Ken met him in 1999 when he was the top government oncologist and president of his medical association of the Mexican state he resided in. Today he continues to run Ken's last open office that administers SEF Immuno-Chemo.™ For obvious reasons, I will not disclose the exact location or his name or the names of the personnel working there. Ken still sends people there who apply at Berkeley-Institute.com.[5] It was this office that first incorporated SEF Immuno-Chemo's™ secret ingredient to nurture the will to live, Tender Loving Care.

# 33

Ken first met this Mexican oncologist through a series of false starts. Between 1992-93 four oncologists in Berkeley signed on to witness and assist in the treatment of a hopelessly sick lung cancer patient. The man had consented to receive SEF Immuno-Chemo,™ but unfortunately died before the treatments could start. Several years later a doctor in Mazatlan wanted to use Ken's artificial liver to treat a patient, and through him Ken was introduced to a gynecologist who had a patient dying from cancer. Again the person died before any SEF™ treatments could start. The same gynecologist mentioned Ken's work to an oncologist he knew. He told Ken the oncologist was very interested in meeting someone who could solve the side effects of cancer treatment. Finally in 1999 Ken met the doctor who would become his valuable cohort. He was a doctor with superior expertise in his field and with a gentle demeanor. The Mexican oncologist spoke softly in excellent English. He told Ken he worked so hard to make his patients better, but he found the side effects from the treatments made them more sick. Ken listened to him. He could see he really wanted to help his patients. Like Ken, it was obvious, he worked from his heart.

Working with this oncologist, Ken continued with more clinical trials. Between 2001 and 2005 they did safety studies on people to make sure no one died from the treatment. Efficacy studies began in 2005 and continued through the middle of 2006. The 2005-06 trial would concentrate on safety, dosage, timing, and efficacy. Four patients consented and were enlisted for the trial. The Mexican oncologist chose two of his own stage 3 lung cancer patients and one stage 4 breast cancer patient. Ken brought in a patient from the U.S. with leukemia. All willingly committed to the protocol of the clinical trial. The hospital administrator, where the Mexican doctor worked part of the time, generously donated a private section of his facility for their use. All four trial patients had received a prior terminal prognosis. They all reached remission within six months and were released from active treatment within a year.

Felicia, a 53 year old woman, had stage 4 estrogen receptor sensitive breast cancer. Prior to starting her SEF Immuno-Chemo™ treatment she received three different standard chemo protocols, but her liver metastasis remained unresponsive. She faced death within months. After four weekly SEF™ treatments, a CT scan showed all her liver metastases gone. Ken and the Mexican oncologist decided to continue SEF™ for another 4 cycles, a total of 8 weekly treatments. Felicia remains alive today, 18 years later.

Jose, a 61 year old man who had lung cancer had received radiotherapy before starting SEF Immuno-Chemo.™ The Mexican oncologist advised that he receive the chemotherapy typically given for lung cancer — carboplatin and gemcitabine on the first day and gemcitabine again on the eighth day after that. This was repeated every three weeks. The only difference would be including mesna shots before and after the carboplatin infusion to remedy carboplatin's side effects. When they tested Jose at 24 weeks, after 8 treatments, he had reached remission. He remained in remission for 8 years before he died in a car accident.

Jorge, a 64 year old man had lung cancer and had been treated conventionally, but was not in remission. After receiving 7 SEF Immuno-Chemo™ treatments over 21 weeks with carboplatin and gemcitabine on the first day and gemcitabine on the eighth day, a clear CT scan and x-ray showed no cancer. He was in remission. He asked to be excused from the trial because he lived 500 miles from the clinic. Ken excused him, and Jose remained in remission for 36 months before he died. At that time 36 months was about two years longer than the average lung cancer patients lived who had received conventional chemotherapy only.

Ken doesn't have a set number of treatments to reach remission. It is a question he is constantly asked, and he routinely explains that results are only as accurate as the test is reliable. But because SEF™ patients don't have to endure side effects, he encourages his patients to continue their therapy for several cycles after tests show their cancer has stopped growing or their tumors have disappeared.

The fourth patient Rose, a 63 year old woman, was getting a blood transfusion every week to manage her leukemia. Cancerous leukemia cells were so prevalent in her bone marrow that there was no room to make healthy red blood cells. She was also on a diuretic to deal with her pulmonary hypertension, a second fatal disorder. Due to the diuretic she was dehydrated when she received her third weekly SEF Immuno-Chemo™ infusion, and her dehydration caused carboplatin to remain in her system unusually long. This extended period of active cancer killing by carboplatin, coupled with mesna protection of her good cells, totally eradicated her cancer. She was able to forego all blood transfusions and remained cancer free for the next 18 months before she died of hypertension.

It may seem that four patients plus Miriam and Sharon are not a large enough sample to "prove" a medicine. However, when results are 100% positive and side effects minimal to none. It is unethical to design studies that use a placebo and not make your therapy available at least on a compassionate basis to the general public.

Ken was encouraged when x-rays showed that breast cancer liver metastases had been liquefied in his in-law. And now with positive test results from his clinical trial in Mexico, he decided to begin treating the public. He started Google ads in 2006.[101] The ads cost on average about $2,500 a month and continue to run today.

Expecting an increase in patient count, Ken's Mexican oncologist hired a young medical doctor, and that doctor hired a nurse. All speak excellent English and have been extensively trained to administer SEF Immuno-Chemo.™ Their standard of care means all staff participate in making sure patients receive the necessary medications, appointments, and appointment reminders. They all do daily charting and reporting, and when necessary go on house [hotel] calls. The Mexican oncologist performs needed surgeries. All regularly consult with Ken. Everyone focuses on giving what is needed, even if it's for basic living and not connected with cancer. At the Mexican clinic SEF Immuno-Chemo's™ special secret ingredient, TLC, a natural part of Mexican culture, and a critical part of SEF Immuno-Chemo's™ treatment, was perfected and has proven vital in saving hopeless patients.

## 34

Ken's Google ad targets patients who have either been dismissed by their oncologists as hopeless, or have quit conventional chemotherapy or immune therapy on their own. Therefore, many of Ken's patients have received extensive amounts of conventional chemotherapy, radiotherapy, sometimes immune therapy or all of the above. Those who resist hospice and/or death by morphine seek alternatives. Some find SEF Immuno-Chemo™ on their own. One oncologist was referring his late stage 4 patients to Ken, and they were responding well. Ken wrote him a polite email detailing the success SEF™ was achieving with his former patients. He also suggested that he release the patients before they were quite so advanced. Subsequently, the oncologist ceased all referrals and correspondence.

People who were either adverse to Western medicine or had witnessed loved ones suffering from standard cancer protocols also inquired. Because these SEF Immuno-Chemo™ pioneers had not been subjected to conventional chemotherapy, radiation, or immune therapy, their immune systems and neutrophils were not damaged. Without the long term side effects from conventional treatments they usually reached remission faster than those who had already suffered through insurance subsidized conventional therapies.

## 35

Besides directing his advertising towards hopeless patients, Ken discouraged people who applied for SEF™ when he thought their cancer remission attainable using conventional methods. If they adamantly refused the toxicity of other therapies, he would reconsider. Ken also tried to minimize the threat his therapy posed to conventional oncology by creating a new field of medicine. He coined the word onsozology.™ Onsozology is derived from two Greek words. "Onkos," used in the word oncology, refers to a swelling or a tumor, and "SoZo" means "to save, to keep safe and sound, to rescue from danger or destruction, to save one from injury or peril, or to save a suffering one from perishing. In essence, saving one from suffering from a disease, to make them well, heal them, restore them to health, or preserve someone who is in danger of destruction."[102]

Doctors who treat only patients who have cancer are by definition oncologists, but Ken prefers to call himself and his associates onsozologists. Credentialed oncologists have three additional years of medical training giving them a board certification in Oncology.[103] They need three years to learn the cornucopia of chemo drugs pharmaceutical companies supply. Because SEF Immuno-Chemo™ does not allow cancer to become resistant to a chemo agent there is no need for so many agents and training time can be reduced. Ken expects both general practitioners and nurses can be trained as onsozologists.[SM] They will need possibly two years of supervised experience to prescribe and administer the dosages necessary for SEF.™ They will need to understand the required scheduling of antidotes with their respective chemo agents, and become familiar with how CT and PET scans, x-rays, Ultrasounds, and blood test results look after SEF Immuno-Chemo™ treatments. They will need to be aware of what reactions to expect from their patients. Of course, they will have to learn and commit to giving their patients' the necessary TLC they need for support.

The onsozology.org[SM] website explains the philosophy of this new medical field. It also contains critical information from popular peer reviewed publications like those from *Lancet* and *New England Journal of Medicine* to help a seeker make informed decisions. It answers the questions people have as they plan their lives after a cancer diagnosis. It doesn't avoid negative research disclosing why conventional therapy is implausible and the pain not worth the result. Onsozology.org consolidates quotes respected journals are willing to write that oncologist don't always tell their patients – quotes such as this one, published in the 2014 Journal of Clinical Oncology, "It seems many patients are not told of the poor expected outcome by their oncologists...86% of patients who undertake a standard cancer therapy do not know it would not put them in remission. Some even thought it would cure them."[104] The article elicits a basic question. Would lung cancer patients submit to conventional chemotherapy, with its life-altering miserable side effects, if they truly realized they would likely gain as little as a few months more of life."[105] Or would they concentrate on enjoying – Every . Single . Day – until cancer killed them? Without accurate, clear, and gently framed information from oncologists, patients are left on their own to decipher and decide the complicated terrain of alternative and conventional possibilities.

Be assured, no one has the time once cancer is discovered to study and create their own cure. It is simply arrogance and panic to try. Ken has spent 65 years and hundreds of thousands of dollars researching all conventional therapies and inventing SEF Immuno-Chemo.™ The last twenty of those years were needed just to unlearn what he expected would happen and understand how SEF™ is different from what's being done.

## 36

After 9-11's terrorist attack, the US government became stingy in granting travel visas into the United States. Even British subjects, Norwegian and Greek citizens would only be granted brief visas and had to return to their home countries to renew them. Mexico, on the other hand, economically depends on tourism. International patients and their supporting relatives found Baja Mexico easy to access and where they could renew their visas. Patients flew into Mexico City first and continued on shorter flights to the clinic. The local community in the small town where Ken's SEF Immuno-Chemo™ clinic is located was looking forward to a new era of prosperity. Ken told me, 18 years ago in a cab ride from San Diego to the clinic, the driver excitedly told him, "A famous doctor is coming to open a cancer clinic in my town. They say the therapy is so good people will be coming from all over the world." I hope during this time of disdain and mean-mindedness towards other countries that somehow, somewhere, this man remains faithful and excited, and that in a small corner of his heart, he still anticipates good times to come.

In 2006 patients trickled in from the Google ads Ken ran in several English speaking countries. Inquirers were told it was a new promising therapy, and they should not give up hope even if they were diagnosed with a terminal cancer. This was not a trial. Ken charged between three and four thousand dollars per treatment. A Bulgarian in his 60s from South Africa arrived in Mexico with late stage 4 colon cancer. But after 8-9 months Ken sent him home. His cancer had responded, but was deemed too wide spread to achieve remission. A Japanese-American business man from San Diego came with stage 4 colon cancer; again there was response, but he hadn't reached remission before he left four months later. Finally, a hospital administrator from Norway, with stage 4 colon cancer spread into his lungs and liver, achieved remission in one month with two treatments.[106] That was more what they had hoped for. The administrator continued for 6 more treatments to waylay any concerns that the conventional cancer tests could be wrong. At a two year follow-up his colon cancer had not returned.

After Ken opened his Berkeley office in 2015 some also came to the U.S. to meet with or to be treated directly by him. But after President Trump's imposed ban in 2016 on people with ancestries from Muslim nations it became difficult for international patients seeking medical care to enter the U.S. One young engineer arriving from Australia, with Australia citizenship but Iranian ancestry, came to Berkeley for treatment. She left Berkeley to visit her aunt in Canada, but found herself blocked from re-entering the United States. Fortunately, at that time Ken still had a clinic in Toronto, so she was able to go there, and didn't miss her scheduled treatment. Later, after sorting out the differences, she re-entered the United States and reached remission at the Berkeley clinic. After returning home to Australia she got pregnant, and in 2019 we were happy to receive a picture of her family, including a new daughter who was conceived and born after her SEF Immuno-Chemo.™ Not all Muslims who were interested in SEF™ fared as well. An Indonesian father was unable to get visas for himself and his eleven year old son who had glioma or brain cancer. The father tried so hard. It tears my heart even now to look at his carefully organized correspondence describing the failed attempts made in Singapore to treat his son. SEF™ was their last hope, and the U.S. visa system under Trump stopped it.

## 37

Some see life as comprised of random fortuitous and unfortunate events. I suppose I felt the same way, though I never forged a plan that would garner me more of those good events. I simply landed where my personal determination to support myself and survive took me. My parents never pushed me to get married or give them grandchildren. They stressed becoming independent. I think their parenting responsibilities weighed heavily and may have inspired that goal. My mother repeatedly told me "don't wear out your welcome" when I'd head out to visit friends, but stopped that admonition after I left home permanently. Raised a Catholic, I left the confines of the doctrine when I was 18 and didn't feel a need to recover. I simply was not up to their standard. It wasn't my fault; God messed up. For twenty years I remained indifferent.

Then life hit me with an emotional knock-out punch, and I broke my own heart. The opportunity wall proved too high for my stunted emotional self to scale. It was accepted and common in the 1950s to stare and make fun of people who were different. I didn't understand it at the time that the whispered ridicule I overheard of my mother's handicap when I was very young chained me to random people's opinions. Years later, a cerebral palsy victim while being interviewed on TV clarified my problem when he said, "The most hurtful part of my disease is being ostracized." I loved my mother, but my linkage to her embarrassed me. I'm not a raving beauty, nor do I primp, but from a very young age I craved acceptance and wanted to distance myself from anyone who might not have the "in" look. I was too anxious to abide by Khalil Gibran's wisdom, "...think not you can direct the course of love, for love, if it finds you worthy, directs your course." Because of my prejudice, I was unable to recognize love when he found me. The years of my life would double before I became whole again.

In an online talk, David Brooks[107] said, "You have to stay in the pain long enough to learn what it's suppose to teach you." Months later grief took me to a level of humility that allowed me to sincerely cry, "God – help me." Immediately, the room flattened as though it were a two dimensional photo, and a stunningly beautiful white crystalline light shimmered about 6 feet in front of me. It was small, about the size of my thumb, if I were to hold my thumb up in front of my face. Like a keyhole to another world, there were people beyond it partying, laughing, and being joyous. Inside my head, behind my left ear, and independent of my thinking, a voice said, "Just don't feel alone." I'd heard this inner voice before, but paid it no mind. Now, by simply asking, it gave me the comfort I needed.

It was the early 1990s when I went to visit my Grandmother Turner. She didn't live next to Ken and his mother anymore. We ate lunch at a small cafe across the street from her apartment. We chatted. I can only guess she saw my sadness. My smile was too heavy to reach my eyes, and our conversation dragged on as I told her about my forgettable activities. Finally she looked at me, and said, "After Molleen, you will be with Ken." She didn't qualify it as an opinion, wish, nor say it with a sigh of regret. She simply stated a fact. I felt relieved. Though I must say also surprised, to hear such a bold statement, when we both knew Ken was happily married, had a 10-12 year old daughter, and was busy working on several promising projects.

I finally sought counseling and during one of the sessions described the beautiful light. The counselor abruptly got up and walked across her office to get a book which she gave to me. In it was the description of my event. The book cautioned, not to believe, but to expect because supernatural events are natural events that just don't happen very often. So I didn't need to have faith. I could just believe the things that actually happened to me. This idea and my now verified one event made me think there was credence to what I was reading. I questioned if we use all our senses. Just five[108] have been recognized, but maybe we have more. Maybe like a color blind person, we're not seeing all there is. We already know we don't hear what cats and dogs hear. We've invented equipment, microscopes, telescopes, hearing devices, etc., to enhance the senses we know about, but we may have capabilities we haven't begun to imagine.

The book also introduced me to a Guru, a person who teaches from their experiences, and a program that offered a different way of thinking. *Samurai Healer* is not meant to promote my or this Guru's spiritual story. I am purposely not identifying the spiritual path I have chosen. I don't expect, nor encourage you to believe my experiences. You can have your own if you want. I do hope you will kindly tolerate and not judge me for them. I've included them because they're part of my decision making process and have guided me.

Shortly after I read my counselor's book, I decided to go the East Bay Ashram for their introductory program. I left in plenty of time. But traffic was hideous. I crawled along. In driver frustration, I cried, "[Guru's name], help me!" Cars started heading to the exits. I saw one careen across three lanes to get off. Everyone moved aside. I thought, "I need to remember this." The road opened in front of me. I sped up, reached my exit, and got off. To my prayer I added, "and a parking space," and found one on busy San Pablo Avenue right outside the door of the Ashram. Still in amazement (if you know Bay Area traffic you understand) I sat down. The video started immediately with the statement, "There are no coincidences."

Occasionally, my inner voice still communicates with me. I've come to feel it's my heart talking, but my ego is strong, and my courage weak. I still resist its guidance, and it's especially hard when it has to do with money. Once it advised me to help my friend, Aubrey, who had exhausted her financial options to pay off a medical debt. This time the voice came with a knock on the top of my head, saying, "Sell your Tesla stock so you can help Aubrey." I relayed by thought—NO. Again, another knock and repeat "Sell...." My answer—NO! I'm not ready to sell yet. Finally a third knock and repeat. I countered ——NO! I have enough money to help her without selling! The voice was quiet. I told Ken about this strange conversation. He muttered, "I think I'll sell my Tesla stock." Just before the end of the trading day Tesla took a dive. It didn't stop dropping until several days later when I sold my stock. Withdrawing money from my savings, I gave it to Aubrey. The gift stung a bit, but I thought I better follow through. Meanwhile, Ken made a bundle.

When Academy Award winner William Hurt was getting his SEF Immuno-Chemo™ treatments for prostate cancer[109] at the Berkeley clinic, he attended the same Ashram. I asked him once what caused him to follow this particular spiritual path. He told me he had driven a friend to the Ashram in New York. When they got there his friend jumped out of the car and disappeared into the building. He waited around, watching people and wondered what they were all doing. Finally he went inside and saw a list of programs. He decided to attend one on meditation. The Swami spoke softly and led the group into the quiet space within each of us. When he felt they were ready he told them to mentally look up. William turned to me his eyes glowing as he said, "I looked up and saw the blue pearl."

We were very sad to hear William passed away in March of 2022. The Channel 5 news reported that his family said he died of natural causes, then countered their statement by adding he had been struggling with prostate cancer for years.[110] Ken does not know how or why William died. When William decided to leave treatment, he sent Ken a touching farewell letter. William had publicized his successful treatment with Ken. Once William confessed to me it took him 10 years to learn to say the 182 Sanskrit verses of the Guru Gita. I smiled, but didn't dare admit that after 20 years I still hadn't gotten them locked and loaded. Now I say it daily. In it, Verse 122 says "They are liberated in rupa (the blue pearl.)" I've never seen the blue pearl, nor reached liberation. So I can only imagine liberation might be similar to what people call rapture or ascendance.[111] I read liberation can happen before or at death, and I think being liberated must be a good thing. I hope his vision of the blue pearl, and maybe other experiences he had that I'll now never hear about, warranted William his highest reward. I pray he is complete and at peace.

# 38

In 2006 just when Ken had made the decision to expand SEF Immuno-Chemo™ he was in a car accident. He and Molleen were visiting one of their favorite vacation spots in Lake Tahoe when they were rear ended while stopped in traffic. The driver behind them was simply impatient. She gunned it as she pulled right to drive the shoulder. Damage was minor. When I took over his Volvo in 2011 I noticed Ken hadn't bothered to repair the crinkled bumper paint. But three months after the accident, Molleen began to experience the symptoms that in six years would take her life.

Initially, Ken's research on cancer continued. He discovered a flaw in a commonly used chemo agent, methotrexate. When cancer patients are given chemo their liver must be healthy enough to detoxify the poison. But with methotrexate, regardless of the patient's liver condition, blood tests showed some people were able to detoxify the poison while others could not. Some patients were as much as 13 times worse at detoxifying methotrexate than others. A patient who could not detoxify the agent suffered many more side effects. Yet it was standard for oncologists to base the dose of methotrexate only on the patient's weight. Ken designed a blood test to customize the methotrexate dose for each patient by measuring the blood level six hours after they received a test infusion of methotrexate. He created Lab-Act.com and a website to advertise a "service" for oncologists, so each of their patients would get optimum results. In 2007 when the American Society of Clinical Oncology, ASCO,[112] held America's largest clinical oncologists' conference in San Francisco he rented a table to personally promote and enlist oncologists to send him blood samples for analysis. In return Lab-Act would send them a customized dose for that patient. With a customized dose methotrexate would become a better cancer killing agent with fewer side effects. No one inquired, except Dr. Akbar Khan from Toronto.

# 39

Dr. Khan had not attended the conference. He was not an oncologist. And he didn't even know about Ken or Ken's cancer work. But Khan corresponded with an aircraft engine parts inspector in Florida, Robert J. Curto. We think Robert first learned about Ken's work from his Lab-Act entry at ASCO, but we don't know for sure.

According to his son, Robert was inquisitive about everything. He subscribed to Time and Popular mechanics magazines to stay current. If he heard or read anything that seemed interesting he would continue researching it online. If he gained more leads, he'd follow through with the involved parties through emails, asking questions, and replying to them with relevant information and contacts. He was good at connecting like minded individuals so they could further their studies. Robert loved helping everyone no matter who they were. His son said you could always count on him. It was his life's mission to help mankind.

When Robert's sister went through chemotherapy he stayed by her side. That may be what drew his attention to researching other treatment options. He saw how the conventional treatment was worse than the disease, and became passionate about helping cancer victims. He gained his knowledge from such assembled sources that he was able to draw disparate conclusions and unique parallels. Though Ken regularly reads all the journals and reports, several times Robert reported the latest "advancements" to Ken first. Once, Robert alerted Ken that the FDA had just approved eleven cancer drugs with only one extending life more than four weeks, but all costing more than $100,000 per treatment.

After ASCO, Robert started corresponding with both Ken and Khan. Robert knew about Ken's work when NO ONE ELSE did. He told Khan, who offered alternative cancer therapy in Canada, to contact Ken, and suggested the two collaborate. The pairing worked. Ken and I flew to Toronto in 2012 to meet Khan. Ken was so impressed that he allowed Dr. Khan to start offering SEF Immuno-Chemo™ at his Medicore clinic. Between 2013 and 2017 Ken worked closely with Dr. Khan while he treated cancer sufferers with SEF.™

Robert was completely unassuming, and never sought recognition or compensation. He started sending Ken expensive gifts of steaks and chocolate covered strawberries every Christmas. Then one Christmas no gifts came. We checked online, and sadly saw he had quietly died. Our Renaissance man would never hear, first hand, how he had effectively advanced treatment towards ending one of mankind's most cruel diseases. He would never know how huge his contribution was towards accomplishing a significant advancement for mankind.

# 40

Dr. Khan, an alternative medicine doctor and celebrity, regularly gave TV and internet interviews. As is common for alternative doctors, he was not without his own controversies. He had already attracted attention from the Canadian Medical Board for using Oncoblot,[113] a test to determine if a patient had leukemia. It was a new test, and not commonly used, or even known about by most oncologists. Ken knew about it, and had used it when he was a general practitioner at the WOHC. But the board claimed Dr. Khan was treating patients for cancer who did not actually have leukemia. Also the Medical Board chided him on using DCA[114] to treat cancer. They disregarded the ton of positive information published about DCA and claimed Khan was using it without scientific basis.

Many of Khan's patients had received a prior terminal prognosis. On his website Khan dutifully recorded patient response to SEF.™ Unfortunately, patients who go to alternative doctors often leave a therapy earlier than recommended to pursue other alternatives. Dr. Khan reported of the 76 patients he had over the four and a half years he offered SEF™ 66 responded, an 87 per cent response rate. He didn't report remissions, though he wrote Ken that he recently corresponded with the mother of a melanoma patient who had metastasis in the brain. Nine years ago the woman's daughter left treatment before Khan had recommended, but today she is well and doing fine.[115]

Dr. Khan's popularity brought lots of patients, but Khan also made SEF™ visible to oncologists. The Canadian College of Physicians and Surgeons of Ontario constantly wrote and criticized Khan for using SEF.™ They said that he did not have evidence it was safe, effective, or that mesna reduced side effects. They accused him of endangering his patients because he was gullible and willing to believe whatever he heard without proof.

In 2013, a 64 years old female patient of Dr. Khan's with pancreatic cancer that spread to five places in the liver responded spectacularly after four SEF Immuno-Chemo™ treatments. Her image test showed SEF™ had killed four of the metastasis in the liver and half of the fifth lesion in the right liver lobe. SEF™ had stemmed the progress of her pancreatic cancer, and she was winning her battle with the disease.[116] But when she had to go to the ER for an infection her prior oncologist was called to examine her. Her oncologist was incensed that she had left her care and was being treated by Dr. Khan. Instead of marveling at her progress the hospitalist and oncologist relegated her to palliative care and alerted the Canadian Licensing Board about SEF Immuno-Chemo.™

The Onterio College of Physicians and Surgeons ruled that Dr. Khan was not to offer SEF Immuno-Chemo™ anymore.[117] Dr. Khan never criticized Ken. He never talked about his daily correspondence and the exhaustive training Ken gave him. He never showed any data he had studied that Ken had not already made public. He took the fall and was barred from continuing SEF Immuno-Chemotherapy.™ Unable to continue her treatments, his 64 year old pancreatic patient died. Finally in 2023, although he was not offering SEF™ anymore, Dr. Khan's entire license was revoked. In 2015 when this saga began to unfold, Ken opened his own office across from Alta Bates Hospital in Berkeley, California, to give Dr. Khan's patients another treatment location.

Some of Khan's patients did come to Berkeley. But most could not afford the travel cost and time. Besides, Berkeley is an expensive place to live. A group that stayed in Toronto tried to sue the medical licensing board,[118] but it seems they don't hurry complaints from terminally ill people through their system. Patients who did come to Berkeley had to return to Canada for simple tests as their national health care only paid in Canada. Scheduling a Canadian medical test is a grueling, often pointless, experience for patients in need of immediate information.[119] Many didn't return.

# 41

In Berkeley, Molleen's condition continued to deteriorate. She had been given a diagnosis of Complex Regional Pain Syndrome, but Ken thought it was more. There is no known cause for CRPS. In Ken's opinion, Molleen's disorder was of the autonomic nervous system which is headquartered right above the brain stem region at the point where the spine ends and the spinal cord meets the brain. This is the most vital and primitive section of the brain, where it connects to the spinal cord and communicates with the rest of the body. It houses the autonomic nervous system which contains centers that control body temperature, breathing and heart rate. The whiplash Molleen sustained in the car accident must have moved her head forward and stretched the fibers of her spinal cord away from the part of her brain that controls the basic functions of life. Initially, the work to communicate her body's functions was transferred to other nerve strands which were not damaged. But eventually, those nerves simply couldn't keep up the extra workload and gave up. Molleen had to quit her job and stopped driving. The driver of the car that hit them was on assignment for a small photography company. Ken hired a lawyer, but they were not able to connect the small accident to the huge disability Molleen was beginning to experience, and she received only a few thousand dollars as compensation.

Now, although quite disabled, she read and was able to understand dozens of complicated books and process thoughts. But she told Ken all emotions had ceased. Molleen, who used to be the heart and laughter of their large family of extended relatives and friends, told Ken she could no longer feel or give love.

By 2008 Molleen was in constant pain, experiencing speech difficulties, and facing growing anxiety and depression. Ken came home to find an empty pain pill bottle and spilled pills in the bathroom. She didn't die from the suicide attempt. But Ken closed his research lab so he could stay home with her. He started sleeping on the floor next to the bed, so she couldn't get up in the middle of the night without his knowledge. He had to earn a living, and hired two caregivers for the daytime while he continued to work at the West Oakland Health Center, his private practice, and collected rental income.

Within a contract that I cannot understand nor explain, the company that held the mortgage on One ALIN Plaza, Dwight Way was able to force a sale. Ken had to give notice to all his tenants. His income from office rentals had paid the mortgage and then some. Proceeds from the sale paid off the large mortgage he had already used to support his research, and he received nothing more at close.

The October 2008 recession started, and normality gave way to knee jerk decisions by our government. President Obama and Congress met the demands of the banks with a seven billion dollar bail out, but they left main street high and dry. Ken was not *Too Big to Fail*, he, like most of us, was too small to save. The U.S. Treasury expected, wished, hoped, but never demanded banks fund low interest loans to main street with the bailout money. So, of course, they didn't.

They horded our tax money and invested it in interest bearing accounts for themselves. Layoffs and foreclosures became Main Streets' everyday trauma, and our country languished during the prolonged "recovery" from the Great Recession.

Businesses made desperate attempts to stay afloat. The West Oakland Health Center tried to roll-out a new medical record system, but the process was so cumbersome patients couldn't get registered for simple appointments and many eventually stopped coming. Revenue dropped. It became impossible for Dr. Cooper to continue leading the Health Center with more and more interference from the non-medical board of directors. Ken, who was then President of the Physicians, and several other "volunteer" doctors quit shortly after

Cooper left. All were near retirement anyway. Younger doctors had not been stepping up to work for the low wages WOHC offered, so no one replaced them. West Oakland Health Center is now owned by Bay Well Health and is a private medical facility.

Ken turned his entire focus to SEF.™ He again reached out to the drug companies. This time he included the media. But a media representative explained that unlike the other things Ken had invented, things they readily covered, curing cancer was a huge announcement. No one wanted to take on that responsibility. It wouldn't be until 2018 when William Hurt came to Berkeley for SEF™ treatments that the press was willing to risk covering Ken's therapy.[109]

Due to the reluctant media, Google ads became the sole method to reach the public. Though his ads did not challenge the established cancer treatments, SEF Immuno-Chemo™ was likely still seen as too much a threat. The hacking and negative blogging increased. Like cockroaches, hackers and naysayers specialize in hiding and multiplying. Try to get rid of them, and they just get worse. You can't tent and fumigate an invention. So we live with them.

# 42

Ken first contacted me with a Christmas card in 2009. He had taken over corresponding to a few people on his mother's holiday list after her death in 2006. In his card he said he was caring for his wife 24/7 after a whiplash from a car accident. He ended advising me to drive carefully. At my "young" age of 60 I had never heard of anyone being so burdened with responsibility. I replied with a card saying I now lived in Danville, a city only 20 minutes away from Berkeley, and if he needed someone to help, I was available. He later told me out of all Molleen's friends and associates I was the only one who offered. Considering I didn't even know her, he thought my offer even more generous.

Strangely, I was available. I hadn't planned on retiring for two more years when I would have qualified for the full benefit package at the HMO where I worked.  But my boss had different ideas.  In August 2008 after working there 11 years they fired me for non-compatibility with co-workers, poor customer service, lack of training, slow ticket closure, and problem time cards.  This didn't happen in a day.  Starting several years before that August, there had been a gauntlet of performance reviews.  First it was only once a year at my no-raise-again review.  But as the years went by the "advisory" conferences increased.  By 2007, I was obligated to meet with my three male bosses almost once a week.  They would take me into a small room to criticize and belittle my work.  As I completed one Performance Improvement Plan, somehow, I earned another.  They brought in HR who threatened me with the Right to Work law, though it had never been approved in California.  HR used a "software tool" to poll every employee in the hospital and medical building regarding my customer service.  This I found out when one person sent me an email saying she didn't know why she was being asked to judge me.[120]  She'd never met me and knew nothing of my service capabilities.  They also sought my co-workers' opinions who started avoiding me like the plague.  By December, when the HR manager advised me to search my soul because that's where she thought the problem stemmed, I reached my breaking point and went to ER.  ER reported my visit and stressed situation to my primary care physician, Dr. Paul Robbins.  I will always be eternally grateful to Dr. Robbins.  As an endocrinologist he knew the damage stress can cause.  He was also one of my satisfied customers and readily approved a leave of absence.  I got full pay for six months and could breathe.

During that time I became more active in the small spiritual center in San Jose started by devotees of my Guru.  I studied at home to pass a few more of the endless IT tests.  I liked my job, even if they didn't like me.  I wasn't going to go down easy.

On Thursday, two days before my leave was up, I returned to work.  That sent my "bosses" into a tizzy.  But it was good to work for two days before they expected me back.  By Monday I was acclimated and ready for the next chapter.  And it came.  I was just shy of completing my 11th year, so I concentrated on stretching out my remaining days to get that extra notch for my pension. I requested as much vacation as I could schedule, being careful to follow the official two week notice rule. In between vacations my assigned tickets were easy-peasy. I even went to the ticket coordinator and told him he didn't have to go easy on me. I was happy to do the hard tickets. He said he wasn't; he gave out the tickets in the order they came in and assigned them according to who was up next. So I changed out keyboards, and mice, and plugged in printers. I felt my Guru was looking out for me. The "bosses" had to cancel one of their meetings. Even though they didn't admit it, there was nothing to gripe about.

I reached my anniversary. Then, in the first week of August several tickets landed in my queue that took a lot of work. I didn't finish them on time due to a "double-time" requirement my manager had created to beef up his stats against other hospital IT departments. It was well known, even by our customers, that other technicians solved this impossible expectation by simply closing their tickets and telling customers "they would return to finish the work." I refused to do that. I closed my tickets when my clients were satisfied. And I might add, I received many tickets based on the unsolved problems of prior tickets that were closed prematurely. My bosses attacked. They scheduled me for a special Thursday meeting. Then I got jury duty and a low number. For the first time in my life I was picked. Except, the trial only lasted four days. In my prayers, I puzzled, "What was that about?"

When I got back to work they set another meeting date, and in it they terminated my employment. No surprise. I had watched others get fired. We were the lucky ones. Sadly, a father of two toddlers committed suicide. I filed for unemployment.

When the representative interviewed me she asked why I was fired. I gave her their five reasons and told her the length of time I'd worked there. I heard my voice crack when I asked if being terminated would prevent my getting benefits. Gently, she said, "I'm the one who decides that." She gave me the benefits.

Months later, as I became accustomed to my early retirement, I browsed a book store where I leafed through a book titled *This Job is Killing Me.* It described the red flags of a difficult boss and how to handle that situation. Then it gave the hopeless qualities of an impossible boss. My boss had all of those.

Less than a month after my termination the stock market plunged signaling the beginning of the 2008 Recession. The government doubled unemployment benefits, instead of six months it would be a year. When renewal was possible in August 2009, I found that the extra week I had worked because of jury duty qualified me for an additional year of benefits. In August 2010, three months from my 62nd birthday, I was gainfully delivered to the door of Social Security.

## 43

I love rain and cloudy skies. So, when I received a small inheritance in 2006, I bought a simple home in Washington state and planned to rent it until I was ready to move. The real estate market was high and I was afraid I'd be priced out of it. The house had a beautiful water view and landscaping, and I made a spontaneous choice without doing much investigating.

Years before a friend had said that she and her husband bought property on Discovery Bay in Washington. When I heard her words my inner voice quietly said, "I want that." That was long before I paid attention to my inner voice, and I pretty much had forgotten the comment. As I looked at the map after the house closed, I saw the water view was Discovery Bay.

Now, without a job, two mortgages were impossible. I decided in favor of a cooler climate and more rain. I also didn't mind leaving my neighbors. They were a very nice 40s something couple, but the man played base in a heavy metal band. He was always cooperative when I'd go over in my night-clothes at 11 PM to ask them to turn it down. She was another story. It worried me that I'd have to disclose their undeniable presence, but began preparing my old craftsman in San Jose for sale anyway.

The house was near the Diridon train station giving it a 100 score for walking access to every place West of the Mississippi. It's location and cuteness made it a gold mine. I'd been remodeling it for over two decades, using the little discretionary money I had, and investing lots of sweat equity. It still wasn't finished. There were lots of details and the normal 30 years of closet clutter to sort through.

I started with the 8 x 8 foot koi fish pond. The filter system had never worked, and the overpopulation of fish made it a mess. I advertised in the local paper "Free Koi." Two people came and took home four fish. Though the sale had not worked, I noticed there seemed to be far fewer fish. While drinking my morning coffee a few days later, I looked out to see a huge blue heron peering into the pond. Over the next few weeks these giant pterodactyl wannabes entertained everyone in the neighborhood as they flew in and out or waited their turn on the nearby rooftops to dine at their sushi bar. My house was 10+ miles away from the park where they probably nested, but this was the only time in 12 years they had visited.

With the fish pond solved, I went on to other issues. My neighborhood advertised a huge garage sale. But when I read the flyer, I stressed that I'd never be ready in time. A few days later another flyer came. The garage sale was rescheduled. I would have another month to prepare. For the first time in 30 years the city completely resurfaced the street. The city also delivered several free dumpsters and placed them around the neighborhood for a day. I loaded up everything I couldn't sell, recycle, or give away onto a movable worktable and wheeled it two blocks into a bin. No need to rent a truck for a dump run. Due to the recession, the master cabinetmaker who had remodeled my kitchen and his top assistant were available and willing to work. They gave me a great price, and finished all my sundry construction details in one day.

One night the house next door was completely dark and quiet. Hallelujah! A week later a friend stopped by. As we enjoyed a cup of coffee, she mentioned a bad smell. I had smelled nothing. But she started looking around and identified it as coming from the house next door. When we checked the backyard we saw the bedroom window was filled with flies, so we called the police. The wife had keeled over while putting on her make-up. There was no foul play.

An autopsy revealed that she died from Hepatitis C. Her husband was away, enrolled in a drug rehab program. He would be gone several more months.

The open house was scheduled for the first weekend of August. Everything was ready except I still hadn't gotten rid of a large metal workbench. It was too heavy for me to transport and sat at the curb with a "free" sign. I called the garbage company to get an emergency pickup. There was no such thing, but they could come Monday. Hanging up, I walked out the back door and down the driveway as a pickup drove by. There was a water heater in the back, and the passenger window was open. I yelled, "Do you take junk." The answer, "Only metal." I pointed to the table. It felt like my Guru was carrying me to the next phase of my life. That weekend 200 people showed up for the open house.

At the very center of the real estate flier was my bookcase, and centered on it, my Guru's picture. I got one thousand over asking even though it was 2009, the bottom of the real estate market. I wouldn't get the "gold," but I didn't mind accepting the offer from a young family. They told me how their two year old loved the house, how he fell asleep on the sofa while they toured, ran around all the paths in the garden, and loved standing on the little bridge I'd made. They also inquired about the chanting book they saw on the sideboard. On closing day I took down my h-OM-e wall hanging, and left with no regrets.

My house was a gold mine. Once the recession was over, it regained its value plus another million. I wasn't suppose to get the gold. But I made enough on the sale and landed completely debt free, a sensation so phenomenal I wished I'd done it sooner. My sweet sister, Marsha, offered me a basement apartment in her Danville house while I finished a few classes aimed at giving me an avocation. That Winter in California it poured rain almost everyday until June. I love rain. It comforted me as I assimilated my change and prepared for my new life.

# 44

Ken didn't accept my offer of help, but he did contact me again in May of 2010. His email explained what he'd been working on. He's quite verbose when describing or talking about his work so gave a lengthy explanation of SEF Immuno-Chemo.™ I guess, since I am not a cancer sufferer, I was able to understand and accept what he said. It seemed simple and straight forward. Protect good; kill bad.

The panic of being diagnosed with cancer must change people's ability to concentrate and understand. Ken usually has to repeat how SEF Immuno-Chemo™ works multiple times before an inquirer can grasp it. Even patients receiving it continue to struggle with why they should follow their treatment schedule exactly for the fastest easiest cheapest results. I think their biggest difficulty is believing they have stumbled upon a treatment that minimizes or is without pain, and one they can continue until they reach remission. It's probably also hard to believe they have found a physician with empathy who is willing to give them hope.

Ken also asked me if I'd like to meet for coffee.

Coffee turned into lunch at the San Francisco City Club. I felt like a hick from San Jose and had to borrow my sister's jacket and purse. I took BART from Walnut Creek, and Ken picked me up in his very cute baby blue Jaguar. I was impressed. He was nervous and at lunch admitted he had not asked anyone out in over 30 years. He told me about Molleen's accident and her current condition. He decided to ask me out because he felt Molleen would want him to take care of his own emotional needs.

We didn't know each other, and talked about Grandma and his mother quite a bit. I felt attracted to him, but worried we might not have enough to talk about after we exhausted the few memories of our past. On subsequent dates, he was quiet, except when talking about his work. Then he could go on for hours. I was fascinated. I hadn't thought much about cancer. It wasn't a big worry. It had not affected any close family members. Cancer can happen to anyone, but those with a family history are more prone to it. Genetically, their immune systems may not be as able to detect and protect them as easily as people whose family history is without cancer. People who get one cancer are more likely than those who have never had cancer to get a second completely different cancer.

I knew cancer was dreaded and thought it must be very painful. But I learned from Ken, cancer can be stealthy while it grows. People tend to ignore its subtle signs because they're not in pain. If they start treatment that's when the pain comes. It's the treatment that consumes a person's life. He explained his therapy eliminated treatment pain and regularly took people into remission. I thought his explanation of how his therapy worked made sense and felt privileged to know this. It took me many years to understand why the world didn't know about SEF Immuno-Chemo.™

Our conversation opened up on many levels. Politically we were very similar. He didn't fly but made an exception when he flew to Washington to protest the inauguration of George W. Bush in 2001. For that same election when the Florida vote count was stopped, I stayed awake all night and wrote a poem which I sent to Justice Stephens.[121] Neither action made a difference, except to make each of us feel better. I was fascinated with Ken's perseverance. I had been with men who talked big about how the world would be better if this or that were so. They were gripers. Ken was a doer. He had planned and was living his life to change things for the better. I wanted to be part of that.

He elaborated on his marriage and explained that early on he and Molleen had agreed they could have an "open" marriage. Although he had remained monogamous through their 30 years together, he was fine that Molleen had exercised that option. He told me about his daughter, Marjorie, who was an only child and of her fierce loyalty and love for her mother. But he knew his daughter also loved him, and he told me both she and Molleen, if he chose to tell Molleen, would be accepting of whatever emotional support he chose to seek in view of the injury Molleen sustained to the emotional part of her brain. Our relationship grew as he dutifully continued to care for Molleen.

He first told me he loved me as we drove across the Bay Bridge in heavy traffic. Did he purposely choose such a romantic time and spot? I'm not sure. Maybe his love of driving and a fun day away brought on his mood. I did not respond until later. I'm a nervous passenger and was concentrating on the road. Then, Ken didn't know about my unparalleled back-seat driving skills. Now, he definitely knows because I will always voice my concerns when it comes to my health and safety. After all, I'd spent a lot of hard years earning my retirement, and I wasn't going to throw it all away in a car accident. Besides as Driving Associate I'm able to start many fun car conversations to make every trip memorable.

I moved into his mother's house.

Ken continued to work at WOHC and advised his staff at his Mexican clinic. He spent hours everyday spoon feeding Molleen and tending to her needs. Initially, she had been able to sit up for a few hours a day to read. But she soon became unable to turn the page. She would signal Ken through the baby monitor to come upstairs and turn it for her. We devised a magnet and paperclip contraption and for awhile she was able to turn up to 8 pages by herself. Eventually, she became almost paralyzed, and on at least one occasion when she was unable to open her eyelids, she still managed to make words asking for Ken's help.

For three years Marjorie visited two or three times a week often bringing Molleen's first grandchild, Heather, with her. Marjorie told me, although it was increasingly difficult for her mother to speak, she still loved being in the room with her and sat and chatted away as though nothing had changed because she felt nothing had really changed. Even though Molleen could not mentally or physically express it, the caring attention her family gave her showed me that her heart must have been just as big, just as loving, and that she must have still enjoyed basking in her family's love. Though she could not cuddle her grandchild, she may well have connected on a deeper plane with Heather's unfettered nonjudgmental baby love.

Molleen lived for two years after Ken and I made a commitment to each other on August 14, 2010. Her agony ended in late October 2012. Giving Molleen all their tender loving care, Ken and his family had nurtured her and survived the siege of her long

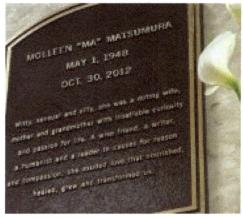

illness. Now missing her became their new pain. A week later a second baby was born to Marjorie's spouse. I'm sure Heath, as any sensitive baby shared in the sadness, but he also brought a bright shining happiness into the little family again.

My transition plan from work to retirement had not started when we remet. It was natural I should be the one to modify my plan. We exchanged commitment vows[122] at the Chapel of the Chimes in Oakland. It's a gorgeous building designed by California's first female architect, Julia Morgan, but it's not the usual wedding venue. We chose it because both his mother and "our" Grandmother are interred there. It was my first commitment at age 61. We went on a one day honeymoon.

It wasn't until 2011, on our first anniversary, that we invited friends to celebrate. Marjorie brought her family. My relatives from Germany and my three siblings attended. Ken and I are not party people, but it was so much fun to share our good feelings with the people closest to us.

We have our issues, but not the problems of conventional marriages. We don't share money, though, Ken is very generous, and I believe pays for more. We don't live in the same house. I was settled at his Mom's and he was settled in the house he and Molleen lived in. Since he likes to work at night and I like privacy in the mornings our hours together became afternoons and evenings, plenty of time to share. I was surprised when I first traveled to my rental property in Washington how I had allowed myself to become dependent. I think dependency can be an enticing slippery slope. So I told myself, "Stop that!" While I think Ken may be a bit dismayed by my independence, it will remain intact, and he'll have to adjust to my need for this source of personal security. For me, our marriage is having someone I can trust who will accept all my thoughts and feelings.

Ken cautioned me regarding divulging our arrangement, saying many people may find it offensive. If you're offended I'm sorry, but it doesn't bother me. As with any prejudice, it only limits you. The powers-that-be who want to stifle SEF Immuno-Chemo™ may find my lack of legal spousal status fertile ground. But my open explanation is simply one of the truths in this book.

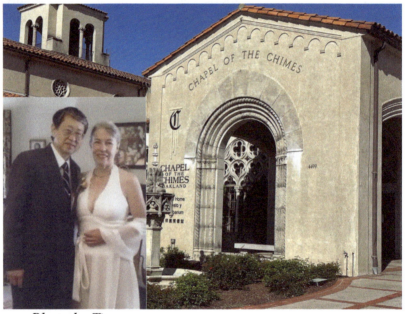

*Photo by Tina
Purpura*

# 45

In 2011 Google ads were working.  Ten patients enrolled in the Mexican clinic at one time, and it felt like success had finally arrived.  But brutal hacking swiftly followed success.  I had worked in a proprietary IT environment and didn't have sufficient network security experience to help.  The hackers were professionals.  At one point Ken was unable to reach a patient.  He called the Mexican hotel the patient was staying at, but was told the patient had checked out.  Only he hadn't.  Ken left a voice mail on one of his doctors' cell phones regarding the dosage for one of the patients.  But she found her vmail full with silent messages and nothing from Ken.  The patient's treatment had to be delayed.  Inquiries from Google ads totally stopped.  When we finally clicked on an ad, we realized we were being ushered onto an identical but bogus website.  Inquiries submitted from it went nowhere.  Against Ken's wishes I created a login for his website so patients could submit and receive secure messages.  Now you can't do anything without logging into a website, but then it was often optional.  My login procedure allowed the patient to submit encrypted information securely onto our server at GoDaddy.  Once there, it would automatically populate a spread sheet.  Ken could open and see all submissions at once.  But no one was applying.  So, with the spreadsheet open on our computer screen, we clicked on his ads, filled out the online Berkeley-Institute.com form with a pretend patient and submitted it.  We watched as the spread sheet populated and the entries just as quickly vanished.  Someone had gotten into GoDaddy's server and added an attribute to each column that deleted any word entered onto that column.  I suspected Ken's programmer, who had suspiciously not setup secondary login authorization, and who constantly argued with me about everything I tried to do.  Ken dismissed my opinion.  He never fires anyone.  But a couple years later the programmer abruptly died from an unknown cause.  Now Ken has a better programmer.

The ten patients in 2011 gave Ken a lot of information about how SEF Immuno-Chemo™ worked, and about how difficult it is to manage people who feel fine.

In conventional chemotherapy patients often feel so ill they continue therapy hoping for the promised remission to end their chemo misery. With SEF,™ patients want to just continue their lives, especially since many are still thinking they will die. This means they want to go on vacations, celebrate every holiday, and attend all their family occasions. Most of the ten patients stayed at the best hotel in the small Mexican city where the clinic is located. They became friends and compared notes on symptoms, progress, and cost. Family members readily contributed to the conversations and ambiance. Being away from home is a huge imposition for any treatment. Boredom began to turn their discussions negative rather then supportive.

The husband of a breast cancer patient decided he should complain to Ken that "Everyone wants to go home." For him home was England, where his wife had already been denied further cancer treatment. The Mexican oncologist indicated he thought she was improving. Her numerous skin tags had vanished and her blood tests supported his observation. Returning to England would mean death. She was only 41 and had three children. Nevertheless her husband convinced her to leave.

Another patient started to get pain in her neck, a location where a tumor had not been found in imaging. She had breast cancer. Her husband thought her cancer must be spreading. After three days the pain subsided. Ken was puzzled. This had not been reported before. After some thought, he realized that the discomfort and the fact that it had subsided was likely caused by neutrophils cleaning up injured cancer cells. He suspected SEF Immuno-Chemo™ had discovered a tumor that hadn't shown up in a prior image and attacked it. Like any injury until the area heals, the pain, itching, and swelling can pinch nearby nerves. Ken realized this was GOOD pain! He tried to convince her husband, whom she had recently married, but the man remained skeptical. Soon after he insisted his wife liquidate her

112

annuity to repay him the money he had spent on her treatment, and they returned to Australia.

Though she quit, her experience gave Ken valuable information. He now alerts all his patients to the possibility of pain in new places, but assures them it will stop in a few days when their immune system neutrophils stop invading the tumor and clear away debris. Being forewarned, they now patiently wait-out the discomfort knowing they're getting better.

A man with stomach cancer received 23 SEF Immuno-Chemo™ treatments totaling 112 AUC of carboplatin, far more than is typically tolerated during conventional chemotherapy. Although it was hard to say for certain, it seemed his cancer had stopped growing. SEF Immuno-Chemo™ is chemotherapy. So Ken initially had his patients check their progress using conventional chemotherapy test methods. But image outlines of known tumors were fuzzy. Fuzzy outlines make everything look bigger, definitely not the result Ken sought. Then he began to recognize that the test results looked more like those expected after immune therapy. It takes several months for the immune system to clean up and heal the area where a tumor has been, so in immune therapy waiting before getting a CT or MRI image is very important.[125] Once the area is cleaned up images again show with sharp outlines of organs where tumors once were, or contain dark spaces [liquified tumors] ready to be expelled.

Ken, like any oncologist, was learning the difference between test results after immune therapy and results after chemotherapy. Trusting the exceptional amount of carboplatin the man had received, his now normal blood test results, including a CTC [circulating tumor count][126] test of zero, and the fact that the patient professed feeling well, Ken decided to release him from therapy. He returned home to the San Francisco Bay Area where as a local musician and entertainer, he started performing again. We were fortunate to see one of his great shows, before his oncologist had their way with him.

It's normal for patients in remission to continue monitoring their condition every few months. So our musician friend returned to his oncologist for his tests. Immune therapy of any kind was still new in 2011, and doctors were evidently unaware that tumor images treated with immune therapy look swollen for months after treatment. They interpreted his CT scans and told him his cancer was worse and all his tumors were bigger. They convinced him that he needed radiation even though they had his SEF Immuno-Chemo™ treatment records, and best practices highly recommend radiation never be done after someone has received extensive amounts of carboplatin.[127] They started and continued radiation on his stomach and throat until his insides ruptured. Ken never saw the man's final medical report, but Ken understands that he was admitted to hospice and died. His obituary said he died from stomach cancer.

Another man thought he could "design his own therapy" and unbeknownst to Ken got infusions of Vitamin C[128] while also receiving SEF Immuno-Chemo.™ His results were puzzling and poor. Large doses of Vitamin C suppress cell division. It is only when a cell divides that carboplatin can kill it or make it sick. Vitamin C slows division, and many people interested in alternative therapies try it. But it doesn't stop cancer growth, and it will never cure it. Once Ken learned of this patients Vitamin C infusions the problem became clear.

Since then, Ken warns all patients not to take supplements without clearing them with him first. Popular supplements such as melatonin, a good sleep inducer, also suppress cell division, and when used during any chemotherapy, melatonin prevents cancer from being killed. Even topical medicines, seemingly as innocuous as dandruff shampoos prevent excess scalp skin from flaking by suppressing the scalp cell division. So dandruff shampoos are also taboo during chemotherapy. People undergoing any type of chemotherapy need to check with their doctors about what they consume or absorb.

A man with colon cancer reached remission. Returning home to San Diego meant returning to his original oncologist for monitoring. Again Ken's patient was told he still had cancer in his colon. He submitted to an operation to "remove" it. During the operation the oncologist stopped abruptly and reportedly said in disgust, "It's full of cancer." The next day family members said their father was doing great. He was able to converse while walking around. But within two days he was dead. Possibly the doctor didn't properly suture the incision, and his patient died of toxicity. The pathology report found no cancer. The family was devastated. Ken tried to convince them to file malpractice charges. But the family, grieving, in shock, and trying to reorganize their lives was too numb to respond. More than a year later they contacted Ken to seek his testimony. But it was too late.

The Mexican oncologist warned Ken that there was a trouble maker in the group. The man liked to stoke negative sentiment among other patients. The patient chose to quit SEF™ before it was estimated he could reach remission. He died a few months after leaving. His obituary said he was a "pioneer in cancer treatment," and he experimented with many therapies for the "sake of others." But I suspect, impatience and negativity were not factored into his supposed study.

## 46

Many patients have had cancer for years before they come to Ken. Often their cancer was not promptly diagnosed, or, if it was diagnosed and they knew about SEF Immuno-Chemo,™ they opted for cheaper or more renown therapies before trusting SEF.™ The more time cancer has to grow and impact vital organs, the greater chance it has of killing its victim. To delay coming and then expect SEF™ to instantaneously turn cancer around is delusional. Ken has had some patients respond and go into remission amazingly fast, but delay gives cancer more of a foothold. It's not going to give up easily. Even in conventional therapy the longer a cancer victim waits to start treatment the more cancer there is to kill, and the more damage cancer can do to the organs it invades.

Once Ken approves a patient who has inquired, he recommends they start SEF™ treatment immediately. Starting immediately and following the protocol exactly means reaching remission will cost less. It also means organs have a better chance of repairing themselves. SEF™ has stopped and eradicated cancer fast enough to prevent organs from failure. Even organs such as the lungs, liver, brain, bladder, colon, and kidneys can repair themselves if cancer is stopped in time.[129] One of the first patients to go to our International clinic in Mexico was a businessman with hepatocellular carcinoma, a liver cancer. The staff found him somewhat brusque and defiant. Before each treatment, he waited until he reached the hospital front entrance before he putting out his cigarette in their planter box. All four quadrants of his liver were in failure. He stayed long enough for his liver to partially repair itself. Once his liver could support him, he quit. The person who referred him to Ken reported he is now doing fine. She said that follow-up doctors found the only cancer remaining was in one lobe of his liver. The other three lobes were cancer free and had repaired themselves. The surgeon removed the bad lobe and he achieved remission.

Making a decision that defies death is, to say the least, traumatic. I'm glad I'm not qualified to describe how difficult it must be. It's hard to break from conventional thinking, unless the patient or someone close to them has had a prior horrible experience with conventional therapy. How can we forge a new path and commit to a decision for such a serious matter? The answer is right under your nose.

Blaise Pascal, a 17th century French philosopher, inventor, and mathematician said, "The heart has reasons that reason cannot know."[130] To me his quote advises us to do diligent personal research, but pause before making any final decision. Breathe deeply, relax, summon the courage to accept the answer, and feel what your heart wants. Your heart will combine your research with wordless reasoning and give you your most sagacious answer. Now you can proceed comfortably and be confident your decision is right for you.

Of course, there are other ways to reassure one's self. Since nausea medicine is available, Ken designs the mesna and carboplatin doses to maximize neutrophil protection then prescribes the same nausea medicine other oncologists use. Since nausea from SEF™ is not as severe as nausea from conventional chemotherapy, one patient told Ken he didn't like taking his nausea medicine because a little nausea fortified his faith that Ken's therapy must be doing something. Strange proof, but whatever works.

## 47

We had hoped the burst of activity at the Mexican clinic would continue with steady enrollment. But it fizzled to one or two then no patients. Google ads still cost over $2,000 a month showing there were lots of people clicking. But inquiries that came through were only from people already too sick to travel, too poor to afford SEF,™ or with difficult family situations. Ken told me he thought hackers were screening his inquiries and letting only the improbable ones through. He spent hours corresponding through email with each person who did inquire. He only corresponds through emails because he finds people often do not understand the first time they hear something. Emails can be reread. With low to no enrollment, it was fortunate Dr. Khan was still able to offer SEF Immuno-Chemo™ at his Toronto clinic.

In 2015 when Ken started looking for office space in Berkeley, I recommended a nurse I knew from the ashram. My ashram acquaintance later told me that she had just updated her resume the night before I called. She offered whatever it brought her as service to God. That next morning she answered her phone and, showing no element of surprise, said I could come pick it up. I gave the resume to Ken to read and retired to the living room. A few minutes later he entered the living room. His mouth hung open. She was incredible and available. She had decades of both U.S. and international medical research experience through the Peace Corp. She also had worked as an ICU nurse at several major university medical centers. Ken contacted her, and she happily joined his staff in Berkeley.

Ken opened his Berkeley office on Colby Street across from Alta Bates Hospital. But Google ads continued to charge for clicks, while failing to supply patients. For three months everyone waited for the first patient.

Finally, Dennis inquired and enrolled in SEF™ treatments. Dennis has been a steadfast advocate for SEF Immuno-Chemo™ for ten years. SEF™ first cured him of terminal bladder and then several years later cured his terminal colon cancer. He shares with us the frustration of SEF's™ delayed roll-out, legal turmoil, and misleading negative reviews. He testified at Ken's trial and was summarily misquoted. He first found the Berkeley-Institute website while sitting in a conventional chemotherapy infusion chair for eight hours. As a software programmer and 49 year old newlywed, he said he was determined to find something better than what was being offered in that crowded chemo room. [131]

After Dennis, patients continued to trickle in from various states and countries. Not as many as TV's Dr. Khan treated, but enough to sustain Ken's remaining two clinics once Dr. Khan was unable to offer SEF™ anymore. Ken's ashram nurse became proficient at the procedure and managed the Berkeley office, while Ken and I started exploring his hope to open SEF Immuno-Chemo™ clinics on indigenous reservations.

# 48

We had often talked about connecting with sovereign indigenous tribes. Ken wanted to give them something to sell other than tobacco and gambling, something that would garner respect with the possibility of making them independent nations again. He thought if SEF Immuno-Chemo™ clinics were available only on their reservations, American and internationals citizens would have to come to native Americans to be saved from their cancer.

Our initial and a consequential contact with Native Americans was Bruce Harris. Bruce's consulting business IARS or "It Ain't Rocket Science" was hired by the HMO I worked for until 2008. He evaluated and scrutinized each technician and the IT department's operating procedures. I easily remembered him because he appreciated my work and even suggested I apply for a lead position. Bruce was also known as Chief Bruce Harris, a member of the Gitwangak community (previously known as Kitwanga) of the

Gitxsan Nation in Northern British Columbia, Canada. Ken and I flew to Vancouver to meet Bruce who would vet Ken to determine if higher level First Nation chiefs might be interested in talking with him. Bruce must have been favorably impressed because we were invited back a few months later to meet with Chiefs Bob and Rebecca Hall of the Stò:lō Tribe of Chilliwack, Canada. Ken spent several hours relaying his story of how his therapy worked, and how and why he wanted to share it with the First Nation and Native Americans of the United States.

*NOTE: In Canada, indigenous peoples are considered members of the First Nation. In the U.S. indigenous people refer to themselves as Native or Indigenous Peoples. It's certainly not official, but for ease of conversation Ken likes to refer to all tribal people of the Western Hemisphere as First Americans.*

Ken explained his intentions starting with his witnessed account of the Washoe tribe about 50 miles South of Reno. He first became interested in helping First Americans when he drove his mother and my Grandmother to Reno to play the slot machines. He never gambled himself because he knew funding his own research made his finances already risky. While they gambled, he would drive to Lake Tahoe and take Polaroid pictures while site seeing.

Passing through Dresslerville, he witnessed the most abject poverty imaginable in the United States. He noticed numerous homes with broken windows, "fixed" only with cardboard or newspaper. Outside the homes littered across yards were beat-up cars and car parts. Inquiring, he was told the blight belonged to the Washoe Indian Tribe.

The tribe had at one time populated the entire Lake Tahoe Basin, Washoe Valley, and the mountain area joining California and Nevada. This quiet peaceful tribe of 1,500 to 3,000 members became known to outsiders in 1844. Four years later when silver was found around Virginia City, Nevada, their life changed drastically. Today, tribal unity is challenged by the very design of their reservation. Homes and businesses are spaced out across a checkerboard of lots separated by properties their non-native neighbors own. The pine groves originally entrusted to individual tribal families for care are now open for pubic and commercial harvest. Tribal members, like everyone else, have to apply for a license to gather no more than twenty-five pounds per household. While the general public sees these expensive nuts as a condiment, for the Washoe people they are a staple. Twenty-five pounds is not nearly enough to sustain a tribal family through a cold Sierra Winter.

The fish of Lake Tahoe and rabbits of Washoe Valley had for centuries given them protein and warm clothes. Now their right of access around Lake Tahoe was extremely limited. It wasn't until 2023 when the ownership controversy of Meeks Bay Resort and Beach was decided in their favor that they regained a piece of the shoreline. The plentiful rabbit supply of Washoe Valley disappeared as parking lots and highways replaced the bush landscape. Progress had not been for their benefit. What his eyes saw made his heart ache, and he thought this isn't right. He wanted to help turn their lives around. But he had just finished medical school on a scholarship, and he was working on a partial salary as a volunteer doctor in America's poorest ghetto. His wealthy father had just sued his mother for divorce. Ken was in no shape then to be helping the Indians. Now was different. Now he had something to offer.

His presentation ended with his intentions. He wanted to collaborate with First Americans by opening clinics on their reservations. SEF Immuno-Chemotherapy™ would not be for entertainment or to capitalize on a bad habit. It would be a life saving necessity. He hoped to hire First American doctors and nurses, but he also knew that locating clinics on reservations would increase opportunities for a variety of supporting businesses. There might even be a possibility that with public demand valuable municipal land might be returned to hosting tribes in order to make clinic locations more convenient for the general public. Ken's medical license would allow him to open a clinic on any tribal reservation land in the U.S.

He thought First Americans probably approached health care in the same holistic caring way as his Mexican staff, and he believed just being exposed to the First American culture would ease stress for cancer patients.

He envisioned the First Americans being treated with respect and appreciation by the descendants of the people who had once slaughtered and oppressed them. He wanted to return pride and self-esteem to all First Americans. He saw SEF Immuno-Chemo™ as a means to lift them out of poverty and make First Americans independent of government support. Fifty years earlier when he witnessed the poverty of the Washoe tribe, he vowed First Americans would be the people his for-profit-towards-public-good foundation would help first. His story and proposal clarified to the Halls the meaning of ALIN Foundation's mission statement, "Bringing tomorrow today. Promoting a Just and Kind World."[132]

Ken's earnest, giving demeanor gained their trust. Chiefs Bob and Becky thought him a man of integrity, and they were interested. But there was much negotiating to do. Indigenous peoples are not inclined to trust. Due to the often barren land they have been relegated to live on, most tribes are dependent. They can't jeopardize the government subsidies they receive. The 574 sovereign nation tribes in the United States and approximately 600 in Canada are dependent on government subsidies. Neither Bruce nor the Halls' tribes were self-sustaining nations.

Bob and Becky had a long history of public service on behalf of the indigenous peoples of North America. They were vocal activists, and met each other in 1976 when incarcerated after participating in a sit-in protesting that the Canadian government return the Coqualeepza property to the 1st Nation. The property had been a 1st Nation school and tuberculosis hospital. After years of negotiating with the Canadian government the property was finally transferred to the Sto:lo in 2023, and it is now reservation land. In Bob's telling of the story he claims Becky chased him until he finally gave in and married her. Becky says it wasn't really like that at all and laughs at his version.

Immediately after the meeting, the Halls started connecting with tribes they were familiar with. Most were in the Pacific Northwest, but word traveled and soon tribes in the Northeast and even Florida

121

were showing interest. There was a major stumbling block though. It seemed Tribal Healthcare services were primarily staffed and run by non-native doctors and nurses. The few indigenous medical professionals the Halls met and talked with were deeply involved in their work and didn't want to risk their careers on a new enterprise. Their hard earned degrees had given them a foothold outside the reservation. No one begrudged them their decision.

By Summer of 2015 it became obvious that efforts to solicit an indigenous staff would waste precious time. Ken had always preferred working with a tribe which would be conveniently located to him. He suggested the Washoe tribe since they had first inspired him and were only a day's drive away. Bob and Becky agreed. They were good friends with a member of the Lummi tribe near Seattle and Chairman Nevers of Washoe's Carson Colony had family in Lummi. Family connection is an important calling card and moves your proposal or issue to the top of any indigenous council's agenda. Bob and Becky, Harley bike enthusiasts, rode the 900 miles several times to visit and establish a friendship and a working relationship with Chairman Nevers and Chief Neil Mortimer of the Washoe tribe. Bob said they especially connected while swapping fishing techniques and stories.

But after much negotiating and several visits, some which included Ken and myself, we weren't able to establish a business partnership. We settled on renting a clean well kept portable building across from their new Senior Center. It had recently been vacated by a government Indian service agency. The tribe would buy the building, and Ken's rent would pay the mortgage plus a bit more. Ken signed the MOU May 16, 2016 and the "Washoe First American Regional Cancer Center" opened Oct. 27, 2017.[133] Our ashram nurse moved into the center area. Surrounding her quarters was a wide hallway with treatment and consult rooms opening off it. The hallway contained a waiting room where Washoe artwork, books describing their tribe's history and it's stories, and plaques explaining Washoe philosophy were displayed. Across from the front entrance our ashram nurse painted a picture of a Washoe family. They stood overlooking Emerald Bay which was once part of the Washoe homeland on the Southeast side of Lake Tahoe. Besides being an excellent nurse and now an onsozologist our ashram nurse has Lokota and Ramura ancestry, and is a certified Cherokee. She was a good fit for our first tribal endeavor.

It was a devastating blow to lose Chief Robert Hall. His ailment was not clearly identifiable. But it was vicious. He became suddenly ill and died within six months. Ken and I traveled to Chilliwack, Canada, for the funeral. He was the Stò:lō tribe's Siyamo'ten, meaning a wise leader and one who cares for others. Chief Bob was buried in the Skowkale tribe's ancestral cemetery in Chilliwack. His grave was dug with shovels. We all filed by adding a handful of dirt before it was closed by tribal members, again with shovels. They had community; they didn't need backhoes. As he was being laid to rest other tribal members played hauntingly beautiful Stò:lō drums. His absence will be a wound that will never close.

In May of 2019, Ken felt a need to recognize and establish Chief Bob's legacy. He invited Becky and her family to the Washoe clinic so we could honor their patriarch by dedicating all future "First American Regional Cancer Centers" to Chief Robert Hall.

Ken and I didn't return for the memorial July 20, 2022. COVID was in full swing. It was unwise to take a chance at being infected or infecting someone else. We sent a video, and in it Ken

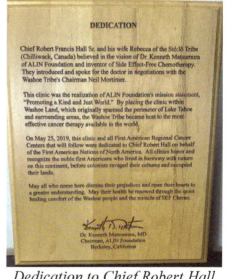

*Dedication to Chief Robert Hall*
*see endnote 136*

expressed his appreciation and admiration for Chief Hall. Chief Becky played it for those who attended the memorial.

For the first two to three years our ashram nurse treated patients, tended to the needs of the clinic's upkeep, and made friends with many of the Washoe tribe members. When asked, she helped them if she could. But when COVID hit at the end of 2019 the tribe decided it was in their best interest to close their reservation to all outsiders in order to protect tribal members, especially the elders with whom our ashram nurse ate lunch with everyday.

Our ashram nurse continued to live in the Regional Cancer Center, and Ken supported it with income from his Berkeley clinic. He hoped to reopen once the threat of COVID passed, but by 2022, with the California Medical Board breathing down his neck, he asked his office staff, contractors, and ashram nurse to start looking for other employment. Fortunately, as the pandemic ebbed lots of jobs materialized, and though he supported them during their search, all sought and found new employment. Sadly, for the second time in half a century (the first being when Molleen was ill) ALIN Foundation was downsizing.

## 92% Long Term Remission of Terminal Cancers

As I previously mentioned the three key terms that describe the outcome of any cancer therapy are response, remission, and cure. I also reported that many SEF Immuno-Chemo™ patients never reached remission for various non-medical reasons such as financial, inconvenience of clinics, lack of family support, prior conventional cancer treatment damage, interference from hospitalists, oncologists, surgeons, and negative stressful thinking. But there is another new reason for a death not due to cancer. One patient of Ken's with terminal pancreatic cancer had started two months prior and was responding well, but he had not reached remission when Ken lost his license. His SEF Immuno-Chemo™ treatments were ordered stopped. Kudos to the California Medical Board and Judge Juliet E. Cox for killing him.

When Ken gave me the following list of remissions for SEF,™ he said he kept it short. He limited his criteria to the pool of patients that (1) he had directly treated (2) who were considered hopeless and who started SEF™ between 2015, when he opened his Berkeley office, and June 2021. I detail these ten later in this chapter. He didn't include patients who chose SEF™ to avoid the toxic side effects of conventional chemotherapy if it would likely have been successful for them anyway. Nor any patient whose treatments began after June 2021, even if they were terminal and are currently in remission because he didn't feel their remissions were long enough to be remarkable. He considers remission successful when a patient has remained cancer free 5 to 10 years, or they've exceeded, by a considerable length of time, the life expectancy for their particular type of cancer. (3) No one was counted who left mid-treatment against Ken's advice, consulted with other oncologists, or were convinced they should continue with and received a different treatment after tests indicated SEF™ had put their cancer in remission.

The 4 patients from Ken's 2005-06 Mexican efficacy trial also fit his criteria (included in the following list and chapter 33) so I added them giving Ken a long term remission rate for terminal cancers of 92%. The only patient on the list who failed had received extensive conventional chemo that devastated her neutrophils prior to starting SEF.™ Even using neupogen (a bone marrow stimulant, commonly used by oncologists) Ken was unable to maintain her neutrophil levels high enough to assist SEF™ in killing her cancer.

I do want to talk about one breast cancer patient age 68 that was not included because she could have survived with conventional chemotherapy. She chose SEF™ instead of adjuvant-chemotherapy plus radiotherapy. As a nurse she was familiar with that alternative. Adjuvant chemotherapy can be toxic and go on for months. Radiotherapy can make breasts hypersensitive and tender to the touch. But with SEF™ she reached remission after only 9 weekly (2 ½ months) of treatments. She remains in remission today 9 years later.

Breast, Patient age 68
Beginning condition: Estrogen/progesterone, Invasive ductal
  carcinoma 6 mm + in-situ ductal carcinoma

Started SEF™ treatment June 2016 Ended treatment August 2016 (9 weekly treatments)

Cumulative carboplatin AUC 14.4

Patient remains in remission today. (9 years)

NOTE: Patient avoided a year of toxic chemotherapy and radiation that can leave breasts hypersensitive to the touch for months.

Around 2018, the pink-ribbon originator, Susan G. Komen Foundation website publicized the conclusion of a UK 15 year study published in 2005 involving twenty-six thousand breast cancer patients.[134] Researchers concluded statistically the benefit gained was 3% greater survival after adjuvant chemotherapy for women aged 61 to 70 who had prior breast surgery. Did these dedicated women who spent so much time, energy, and money supporting breast cancer research really consider these results satisfactory?

SEF™ treatment schedule is not time consuming. Patients come in one day before their chemo infusion for a mesna shot. They return the next day three hours prior to their chemo infusion for another mesna shot. The infusion itself takes between 20 and 45 minutes. Depending upon the AUC (dosage) of the carboplatin (or another chemo agent,) they return the next one or two days to get a mesna shot at each visit. Many people continue working during therapy.

After Ken lost his license, SEF™ success continues at his Mexican clinic. Some of his Berkeley patients, who could afford to go, reached remission there. One patient from Australia started in Berkeley in May of 2023 with advanced pancreatic cancer spread to her lungs and bone. Her case was considered hopeless, especially in Australia a country with national health care, but she reached remission in Mexico and has since returned home. A multiple myloma patient responded well. But traveling from the San Francisco Bay Area to Mexico created extreme difficulty for her. The Medical Board's order added an inordinate amount of stress to her situation. She lost her job and her home. But she is a fighter and persevered. Now, she has returned to Oakland where she continues with conventional chemotherapy.

Science measures new treatment results with mathematics to determine if good results can be repeated or were they're just a stroke of good luck. Mathematical determination is called 'statistical analysis.'

Most new chemo therapies aren't expected to 'solve' cancer forever, only to offer a slight improvement over existing therapies. To statistically measure anticipated tiny improvements, sometimes, as little as 2%, you need to collect data on tens of thousands of patient volunteers. Adding a placebo (sugar pill) or the existing drug the trial drug is being compared to, makes it a "double blind" trial.

*NOTE: A double blind trial is conducted by giving the administering doctor two bottles of identical capsules. One bottle is labeled "A," and the other is labeled "B". Only one bottle contains the new drug being tested. The doctor divides his volunteers into two groups. Depending on your group you receive only the A or only the B pill throughout the trial. No one knows until the end of the trial who got the drug and who got the placebo.*

Just using a placebo means twice the number of people have to participate. It also means, if a sugar pill is used half the group will get no benefit for their time and the inconvenience of being in this trial. Besides the cost drug companies spend to develop the drug, they must also pay thousands of dollars to each university oncologist administering the trial for their time convincing, enrolling, monitoring, and reporting on the patients. When drug companies spend so much money developing and testing a new chemo agent, failure to sell it is untenable. Trials that fail burden other drugs in the company's "pipeline" with their monetary losses. But trials that show any improvement, even 2%, give the FDA reason to approve the drug, and the company is then free to sell it.

Comparing SEF Immuno-Chemotherapy™ which is without side effects, seldom fails, and is effective on multiple types of cancer to ordinary chemotherapy which fails quite often and is toxic just doesn't take thousands of people – like it doesn't take thousands of people to determine if a square of sweet dark chocolate is preferred over a spoon full of flour/water paste.

SEF Immuno-Chemotherapy™ is markedly better because in even the most hopeless cases it regularly takes the cancer victim to long term remission.

The results of the below patients are also published in the online peer-reviewed "Journal of Medicine & Biology." The article by Kenneth Matsumura can be read at endnote [137] or by going online to www.jmbio.org. At the search bar, type Kenneth Matsumura and click search by author name to find the article entitled: *A Novel Immuno-Chemotherapy: Inducing Long-term Remission without Side Effects.* Search with the paper's title to read its peer review.

### Bladder Patient age 49

Beginning condition: 2014 High grade P3 urothelial cancer.
Surgical resection of distal right ureter and re-implantation at Stanford University Hospital. 2015 Recurrence.
Recommended to undertake four high dose chemo and undergo bladder excision, but given a prognosis life expectancy of 1 to 2 years.

Started SEF™ treatment September 2015 Ended December 2015.

Cumulative carboplatin AUC 40

Patient remains in remission today. (10 years)

### Breast Patient age 45

Beginning condition: January 2017 Mastectomy for 2.6 x .8 x 1.5 mass. Poorly differentiated invasive ductal triple negative cancer.

Started SEF™ treatment May 2017 Ended January 2018. 8 individually scheduled AUC 4

Cumulative carboplatin AUC 13.6

Patient remains in remission today. (7 years)

Breast Patient age 51

Beginning condition: 2013 underwent lumpectomy, radiotherapy, chemo to address 2 cm mass in right breast. 2017 Triple negative breast 4.5 cm mass in left breast addressed with bilateral mastectomy, chemo. 2019 Brain parietal lobe metastasis addressed with three surgeries, gamma knife radiotherapy, but resulting in no resolution at Canadian Health in Alberta, Canada.

Started SEF™ treatment June 2020 Ended. January 2021 bi-weekly treatments

Cumulative carboplatin AUC 21.5

Patient remains in remission today. (4 years)

Breast, Patient age 54

Beginning condition: 2015 – 1.6 cm invasive ductal carcinoma triple negative breast cancer. Oncotype score 63 denoting high recurrence risk.

Started SEF™ treatment June 2020 Ended Nov 2022. 32 bi-weekly AUC (mostly) 4

Cumulative carboplatin AUC 129

Patient remains in remission today. (3 years)

Breast, Patient age 75

Beginning condition: Left invasive ductal ca axillary dissect 2017; received adjuvant (ordinary) chemo for recurrence axillary and subpectoral lymph node metastasis 2020. Started letrozole, but condition continued to deteriorate. CTC (circulating tumor count) 1 million

Started SEF™ treatment December 2020 with 4 carboplatin AUC 4. CTC reduced to 250,000. Treated low neutrophil issue caused from past adjuvant chemo with filgrastim to stimulate marrow to produce neutrophils.

Cumulative carboplatin AUC 35 over 10 treatments.

Patient failed. Referred to traditional oncologist, to deal with liver metastasis.

Breast, Patient age 38

Beginning condition: 2014, Estrogen/progesterone receptor positive. Mastectomy for 9 cm DCIS high grade, suggestive of poor prognosis (Endo predict score 4.4, Ki 67-20%.)

Started SEF™ treatment September 2016 Ended treatment January 2017. 7 weekly, 4 biweekly treatments.

Cumulative carboplatin AUC 29.9

Patients remains in remission today. (9 years)

> NOTE: Conventional treatment recommends all estrogen positive breast cancer patients start estrogen hormone-sensitive suppressive medicines. Most become sterile after these medicines. Those who are not sterile are advised not to become pregnant as high estrogen levels during pregnancy could activate any residual cancer cells. But this patient had a three year old son, and she wanted a daughter. SEF™ treatment does not include hormone suppressants. When she reached remission, Ken was confident enough in SEF™ to encourage her to get pregnant. Happy and grateful she delivered a beautiful daughter three years later.

Breast Patient age 48

Beginning condition: September 2017 Estrogen/progesterone plus mass. Had mastectomy only while in Canada.

Started SEF™ treatment immediately after mastectomy. 9 biweekly carboplatin AUC 3.5, 17 carboplatin AUC ≤ 2.

Cumulative carboplatin AUC 65

Patients remains in remission today. (8 years)

## Colon Patient age 53

Beginning condition: Sigmoid colon cancer spread to submucosa, para-aortic lymph node and 3 mm liver lesion.

Started SEF™ treatment March 2019 Ended September 2019. 13 bi-weekly SEF™ treatments averaging AUC 4.

Cumulative carboplatin AUC 52

Patients remains in remission today. (6 years)

NOTE: Ordinary chemotherapy cannot eradicate cancer in para-aortic lymph nodes. They must be surgically removed.

## Pancreas Patient 57

Beginning condition: 2016 pancreatic tumor at head of pancreas; with suspicious liver metastasis.

Started SEF™ treatment August 2016 Ended September 2017. 12 bi-weekly AUC 4; 5 bi-weekly AUC 3.

Cumulative carboplatin AUC 63.

Patients remains in remission today. (8 years)

## Lung Patient age 85

Beginning condition: Non-small cell, 3.5 x 2.7 cm tumor in right upper lobe. 3.7 x 3.3 cm and 1.2 x 0.7 cm in left lobes.

Started SEF™ treatment July 2018 Ended April 2019. 14 bi-weekly AUC 3. Upper left lobe tumor smaller (2.2 x 1 cm) and second left lobe tumor showing no blood flow April 2023.

Cumulative carboplatin AUC 42

Patients remains in remission today. (6 years)

## Breast Patient age 53

Beginning condition: Diagnosed June 2005 lobular carcinoma, Estrogen and progesterone positive. Treated with lumpectomy and auxiliary dissection. Four months later developed a single liver metastasis that was treated with four cycles of capacitabine and paclitaxel without effect.

Stated SEF™ carboplatin weekly treatment December 2005 AUC 2. Ultrasound after four treatments showed liver lesion cleared. Underwent four additional SEF™ cycles.

Cumulative carboplatin AUC 16.

Patient remains well and free of cancer 19 years later.

Lung Patient age 61

Beginning condition: Diagnosed with non-small cell stage 3B lung cancer. Received 20 Gy radiotherapy.

Started July 2005 with standard chemo protocol for 2005 era. Comprising of carboplatin AUC 5 every three weeks, supplemented with gemcitabine on day 1 and 8. Day 8 gemcitabine was omitted with cycle 8. Mesna antidote was added before and after carboplatin infusions. Total of 8 combined cycles of standard protocol with SEF™ mesna added.

Cumulative carboplatin AUC 45.

Patient went into remission and remained so for eight years when he died in an auto accident.

Lung.Patient age 64

Beginning condition: Diagnosed as recurrent non-small cell lung cancer stage 3B. Treated previously, but not in remission.

Started February 2006 with protocol based on standard chemo of 2006. Comprising of carboplatin AUC 5 every three weeks, supplemented with gemcitabine on day 1 and 8. Patient underwent 7 cycles and was granted excused from the eighth because of 500 mile travel from home.

Cumulative carboplatin AUC 35

Patient went into complete remission for three years when he recurred suddenly and died. 2006 life expectancy for non-small cell lung cancer after initial diagnosis was 9 months.

## Leukemia, Myelogenous age 61

Beginning condition: Many years history of myeloproliferative disorder which went into acute leukemic phase requiring weekly blood transfusion due to marrow inability to make red cells.

Started SEF Chemo in September 2005 with 3 weekly AUC 1.6 carboplatin. Because the patient also suffered from pulmonary hypertension for many years and was taking diuretics, she tended to be dehydrated causing anuria, which can result in retention of carboplatin effectively making carboplatin dose of AUC 1.6 more equivalent to AUC 5 or 6. After three weeks, her neutrophil count was too low to continue SEF.™ However, the patient's hemoglobin stabilized without transfusion.

She required no more SEF™ treatments and remained hematologically stable for 18 months at which time she expired due to her pulmonary hypertension.

# Tomorrow

Ken still wants to offer and engage the First Americans of North America to host SEF Immuno-Chemotherapy™ Regional Cancer Centers. He wants the revenue gained from providing this therapy to the world to make them independent sovereign nations. In 2024 Congress allocated only 24 billion dollars to be shared among the 574 indigenous tribes of the United States – not nearly enough to change their impoverished lives. Ken will gather those he's worked with before and follow their direction on how to go forward. With independent First American land checker-boarding the U.S. to conveniently locate SEF™ Regional Cancer Centers U.S. subsidizing dollars will not be necessary. First American countries will be respected trading partners, and hopefully, the injuries from abuse and disrespect for their existence will begin to heal.

According to the World Health Organization worldwide cancer deaths are 10 million. To make SEF Immuno-Chemotherapy™ convenient worldwide Ken is working on taking the treatment offshore by registering vessels in treatment friendly countries that will dock at major ports in Europe and the Pacific Rim.

## During the last 30 years the percentage of people in the U.S. dying from cancer under our current medical system HASN'T CHANGED.

Using advanced arithmetic to do my "statistical analysis."
1990 cancer deaths 473,500 ÷ **1990** U.S. pop 250.1 mil =**.189%**
2000 cancer deaths 553,080 ÷ **2000** U.S. pop 282.2 mil =**.195%**
2010 cancer deaths 569,490 ÷ **2010** U.S. pop 309.3 mil =**.184%**
2020 cancer deaths 606,520 ÷ **2020** U.S. pop 331.5 mil =**.182%**

Cancer has been cured in your lifetime. You simply did not know. Without a medical license, it will be harder and take Ken longer to achieve the success he envisions. Your participation can change that. You can make SEF Immuno-Chemotherapy™ available now for you and for your loved ones.

Call or write to the President of the California Medical Board Kristina D. Lawson, J.D. Ask that the license of Dr. Kenneth Matsumura to be reinstated. Cite case #800-2019-059098. If you do not get a satisfactory reply write to California Governor Gavin Newsom.

## 51

A little over a year ago my brother Paul and I boarded the 8 AM train out of Denver. I hate traveling, so a trip to see our sister was pretty rare. We headed to the train's diner and a French toast breakfast. Per custom, the waiter seated a young woman across from us. I could see she was handsome, but this morning she looked like she had just rolled out of bed. In conversation, I found she had just gotten on too. She grabbed her newspaper, but couldn't read, so left for a moment to get her glasses. When she returned she wore the most artistic, yet stylish and sophisticated glasses I'd ever seen. I think she spoke first. Saying, "Now I can read."

Paul left, and she and I made a few opening comments. I asked her what she did. She chirped something about films, and we went on to talk about family, visiting, and the fact she preferred train travel to driving, even for this short three stop trip. I asked more about her films job. She told me she was a director, writer, and actress. It had only been two months since Ken's license was revoked, and I told her a bit of his story. She leaned forward and asked me if I had started my book yet. I said it was my plan to start as soon as I got back to Berkeley. She seemed excited and said we should exchange contact information. She handed me a piece of paper with her name, Miranda Bailey, Cold Iron Pictures. As she left, she told me to watch some of her movies.

NOTE: *To read endnotes and to see the pictures larger go to Samurai-Healer.com*

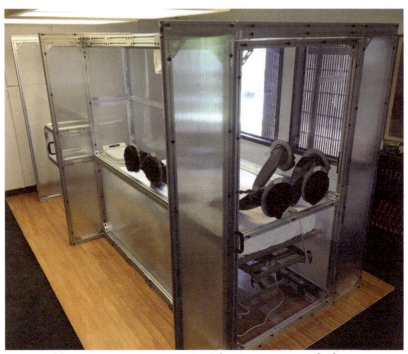

*Negative pressure air inside vents out cooled air through 400 F degree air purifiers.*

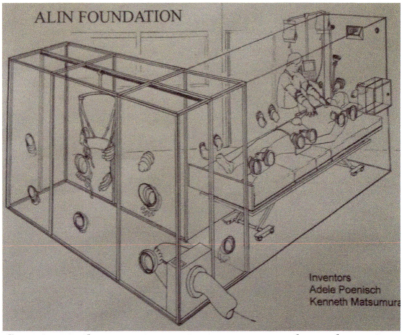

ALIN FOUNDATION

Inventors
Adele Poenisch
Kenneth Matsumura

*Contains: toilet, exercise equipment, can attach to other units.*

# Addendum

I am Ken Matsumura. Adele has been involved with my SEF Immuno-Chemo™ project for nearly 15 years and knows more about SEF Immuno-Chemo than virtually anyone else. I thought that this book doesn't talk enough about one subject, and I asked her to allow me to write this "addendum," since she is too modest to present it herself.

In 2014, when a patient with Ebola arrived in Texas to be treated, our country was not prepared for anything so contagious and deadly. The U.S. had only 8 Ebola isolation beds and expanded that to only 35 Ebola treatment centers before the Ebola threat ended. Two caregivers, a doctor, and a nurse caught Ebola from just the one initially infected patient. Despite such an obvious failure at preparedness, our country took no further steps to ready for the next infectious disease outbreak. Fortunately, Covid-19 was not as infectious and not as deadly.

Adele invented a method/device for containing deadly germs. It is an enclosure that an infected patient can be placed inside. Caregivers administer to the patient through glove portals placed at all critical locations. They do not need to dress in bulky hazmat suits, yet they remain safe from deadly pathogens.

Fatality from Covid was 6 per cent and first responders and medical personnel persevered. But there are some infectious diseases in the world today that have a fatality rate of 50 to 80 per cent. Can we really ask or expect medical personnel to continue serving when it will likely result in their own deaths?

Three years ago the CDC asked scientists to submit grant proposals for dealing with infectious diseases. Adele did, and her proposal was approved, but not funded. It was patented though by the European Patent Office.

We built a prototype and introduced it at a press release. See Feb. 26, 2020 ABC7news.com "New Equipment Developed in Berkeley Could Help Slow Coronavirus Spread and Feb 27, 2020 CBSnews.com "Containment Capsules Provide a Safer Way to Treat Coronavirus Patients."